No one wants to die, alone

When a loved one is faced
with terminal cancer

NICOLE ARMSTRONG

FriesenPress

Suite 300 – 990 Fort Street
Victoria, BC, Canada V8W 1H8
www.friesenpress.com

Copyright © 2014 by Nicole Armstrong
First Edition — 2014

Contributors: Ariane de Bonvoisin
Donald Nadeau: Front cover photograph

Excerpt(s) from HELP ME LIVE, REVISED: 20 THINGS PEOPLE WITH CANCER WANT YOU TO KNOW by Lori Hope, copyright © 2005, 2011 by Lori Hope. Used by permission of Celestial Arts, an imprint of the Crown Publishing Group, a division of Random House LLC. All rights reserved. Any third party use of this material, outside of this publication, is prohibited. Interested parties must apply directly to Random House LLC for permission.

All rights reserved.

No part of this publication may be reproduced in any form, or by any means, electronic or mechanical, including photocopying, recording, or any information browsing, storage, or retrieval system, without permission in writing from the publisher.

ISBN
978-1-4602-5191-1 (Hardcover)
978-1-4602-5192-8 (Paperback)
978-1-4602-5193-5 (eBook)

1. *Self-Help, Death, Grief, Bereavement*

Distributed to the trade by The Ingram Book Company

Author's note: This book is a memoir. It reflects my recollections of events, incidents and dialogue to the best of my memory. Although in some cases dates may be inaccurate, incidents and dialogue may have been condensed, the book continues to convey the essence of what was said or happened. All characters are real. Most names have been changed in order to protect the privacy of individuals. This memoir is written from my perspective and the opinions and views expressed are my own. The intent of my work is not to offend or discredit anyone, it is to recreate as accurately as possible the challenges and opportunities a family may face when a loved one is diagnosed with terminal cancer. The reader is responsible for his or her own choices, actions and results.

In loving memory of Carmen, Robert and Léopold

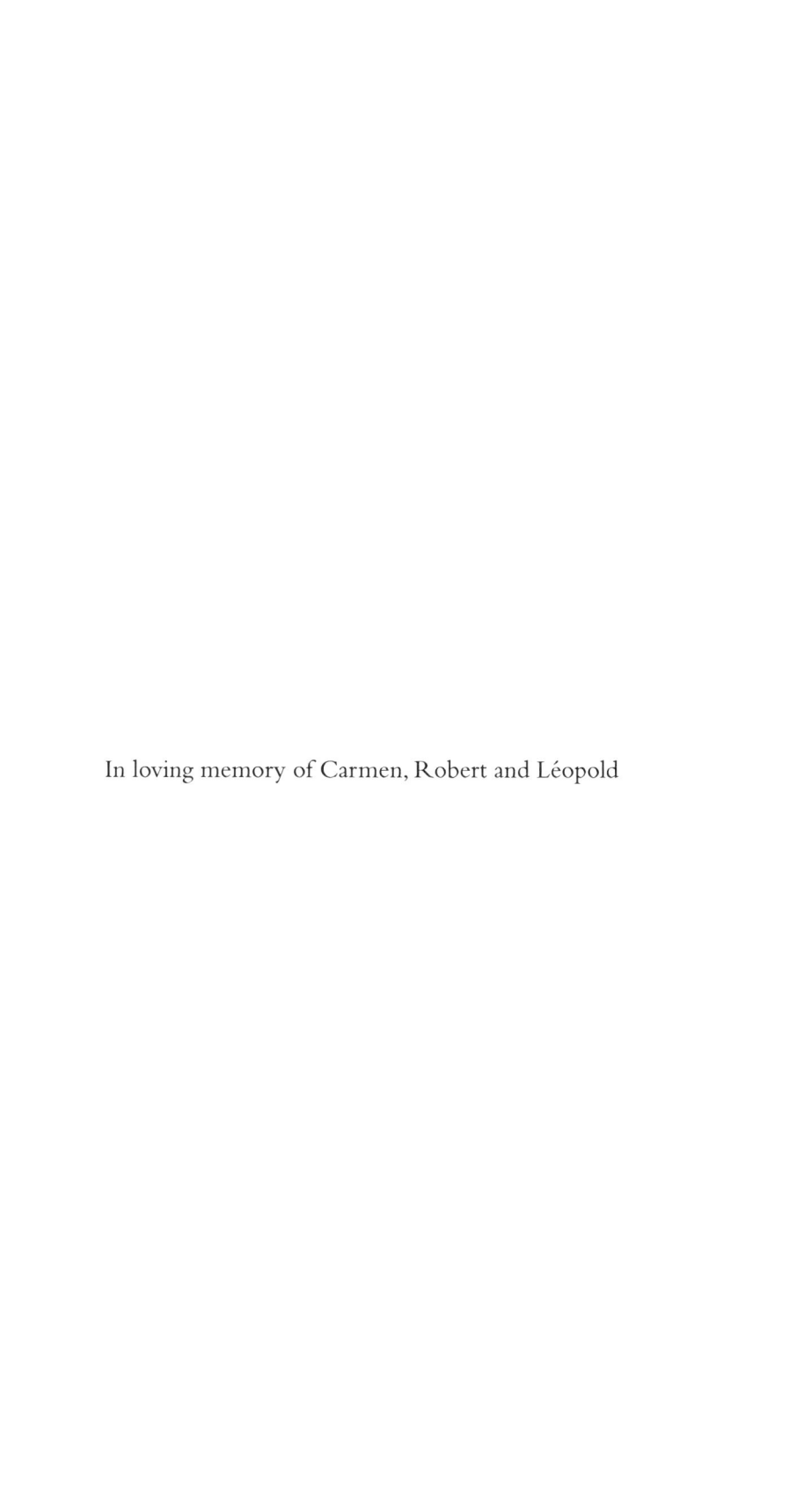

TABLE OF CONTENTS

Acknowledgements x
Special Recognition xi
Preface xiii
Author's Prefatory Note xvii
Introduction xix
The Five Stages of Death xxii
The Five Stages of Family Grief xxiii
Was He Talking to Me? 1
Enough with the Reinforcement 12
Pray for Me I Am Terrified 48
How Can I Ever Thank You? 80
A Constant Battle 92
Travel Plans 113
It's Time 123
Saying Goodbye 140
The Aftermath 152
Writing This Book 160
A Thank You Letter to George 163
Conclusion 165
Special Contribution
by Ariane de Bonvoisin, Change Expert 167
Afterword 172
Other Readings 174

ACKNOWLEDGEMENTS

Thank you to all who have written books on the topic of death and dying, surviving cancer, guides to coping ... it helps us poor lost souls in dealing with our challenges and supporting our loved ones.

Thank you to all health care providers who take a moment to care and show compassion. Thank you to those who understand the value and role of family: especially at the end of one's life.

Thank you to all volunteers. It matters.

SPECIAL RECOGNITION

There is goodness in people. Many wonderful individuals have been helpful to me in writing this book.

I appreciate the support of friends who acted as a sounding board on many occasions.

I am particularly grateful to Dr. Steve Pelletier, Margaret Dukes, Debbie Bolger-Ingimundson and Lucie Guimond for their time and willingness to review an early draft of my manuscript. Their different perspectives and candid feedback encouraged me to pursue my plans to publish this book. Thank you for believing in this project.

I extend a heartfelt thank you to my editor, Janet Love Morrison, for her generosity and guidance.

I am honoured and privileged to have the company of Ariane de Bonvoisin in my memoir. Thank you for your generosity and for inspiring us with "The 9 Principles of Change."

I am blessed with a special family. I offer them all my love and gratitude. Thank you for allowing me to share our story.

To Gérald, my loving husband and soul mate – thank you for never asking me to choose between our relationship and my support to my family. This book would not exist without your love, your continued support and encouragement.

Last but not least – thank you to my dearest sister Carmen. I use your words when I say – I love you with all my heart. Your best friend, bosom sister forever and ever.

PREFACE

I write this book for many reasons: To find myself, to educate and help others who may be struggling in the same way, and in memory of my sister.

I share with you our most intimate year in hope that it may assist you and others to help your loved ones and yourself.

Losing someone you love to terminal cancer is heartbreaking. Sharing their journey is challenging in all aspects: it alters your life and brings emotional, psychological, physical, financial and family issues to the forefront. You may face barriers with the health care system and pressure from health care professionals. You will meet health care providers who are caring, and others who lack compassion and understanding of end-of-life issues. Complexities related to processes of employers and insurance companies and the various bureaucracies exacerbate an already difficult situation. You live with death and grieve the living. You don't know when it will end. Regardless, you are not ready.

At times, you feel people can't relate – that they don't understand. People are uncomfortable talking about death and the terminally ill. Many feel awkward talking with the dying. Others can't psychologically deal with life-threatening situations. And some don't know what to say and do, they stay away. While others support you the best way they can.

Yet death is another phase in life, one that is inevitable, one that is much bigger than any of us. It is a phase unknown to most of us until it reaches our being, until it reaches a loved one. All too often, it arrives prematurely in our lives. It takes us outside our comfort zone and introduces end-of-life issues with intense and powerful emotions – you learn as you go.

Death for the terminally ill is not an event but a process. Many don't fully realize the challenges and opportunities involved. This will most likely change. As the baby-boomer population ages, more people will face terminal illness. More will become caregivers. More will experience intense loss.

In the book *Saying Goodbye – A Guide to Coping with a Loved One's Terminal Illness*,[1] the authors identify how death and dying have dramatically changed thanks to medical advancement. Sudden death has become less imminent and is replaced with a terminal diagnosis, sometimes with a prognosis of many years. With this, the so-called traditional grief is being replaced with a contemporary one, one they refer to as – the new grief. This prolonged grief brings new and complex challenges for the family and patient.

I came across this book late in my sister's journey. I found the authors' introduction of the five stages of family grief quite pertinent: Stage 1 – Crisis; Stage 2 – Unity; Stage 3 – Upheaval; Stage 4 – Resolution and Stage 5 – Renewal. This new grief is real. It is confirmed by my family's experience. The stages of family grief become evident as my story unfolds.

Another treasure is *Help me live – 20 things people with cancer want you to know*.[2] This great resource helps you to understand what patients with cancer are living. A summary of many chapters is intertwined in my book. My summaries have brought a common dialogue amongst our family members and friends, and it helped us be there.

On occasion I hear, "I'm not afraid of dying." Easier said when death is not at our doorstep. Perhaps what people fear is not death itself but the process of dying – when physical limitations set in, the disability, the loss of independence and the suffering. Perhaps the focus is being ready to say goodbye to your loved ones and in letting go of your life on earth. Perhaps the fear is of so many unknowns.

Cancer is the leading cause of premature death in Canada[3] and the second most cause of death in the US.[4] Every day, close to 1800 people are expected to die of cancer in Canada and the US alone. How will

---

[1] Okun, Barbara and Joseph Nowinski. *Saying Goodbye: A Guide to Coping with a Loved One's Terminal Illness*. New York: Berkley books, 2011. Print.

[2] Hope, Lori. *Help Me Live: 20 Things People with Cancer Want You to Know*. New York: Random House, Rev. ed., 2011. Print.

[3] http://www.conferenceboard.ca/hcp/details/health/mortality-cancer.aspx (accessed May 24, 2014).

[4] American Cancer Society, Cancer Facts and Figures 2014. Atlanta: American Cancer Society; 2014.

you support your loved one on their journey? Can such an experience be enriching?

How you contribute to a good death is your choice. You may not understand what your loved one is going through. You probably never imagined yourself on a death bed or living a death sentence. But what if it was you? What would be important to you as a dying human being?

Imagine a change in your life's priorities. Imagine the opportunity to offer the greatest gift of love. Such a journey involves the people who are important to the dying. It involves you, family and friends, and it involves your loved one. Death is not an individual but a family experience. Deep within us we find the courage to help our loved one and we learn to forgive. It can become the most caring and compassionate thing we do.

AUTHOR'S PREFATORY NOTE

This is my story.
It is written from my perspective, my reality.
It is written with love.

As you turn this page, you enter my life and my family's.
I invite you to read this book with an open heart
for there is no space for judgment.

INTRODUCTION

I don't know what brought me to write my first few paragraphs. These were written at the very beginning of this family crisis. They were forgotten for months until it became evident I needed to journal to manage my stress and retain my sanity during this emotional and heartbreaking episode of my life.

To witness and accompany someone you love dearly on their journey to the next world is a choice and a privilege, and by far one of the most challenging emotionally and psychologically. One can easily get lost in the turmoil. You mourn from the day you hear the drastic news and it continues beyond the funeral. It can easily become chronic.

I return to writing this book, days after my sister's passing. Initially I thought it would be my gift to her but it became extremely difficult emotionally. I was reliving the past year all over again but this time retrospectively. If only I had known. Today I complete this book because there is no return. Could it be a call for understanding?

Sharing my father's journey was one of the most enriching experiences in my life: sharing my sister's was totally different. Although there were similarities, our close relationship as sisters and friends made it unique and difficult to let go. It continues to be surreal.

Upon her passing, I was tormented with feelings of guilt, selfishness and shame. I believed I abandoned her during her last days. I sought comfort in reviewing our emails. Particularly the ones where she would thank me for helping her and tell me she loves me.

I struggle to understand my emotions and the different stages of my mourning. Sometimes I can't even bring myself to look at her picture, or to call her name aloud. Other times, I was upset with her children for what I perceived to be their lack of contribution and dependency. Why was it so easy for them to let go?

My feelings are based on my perspective, my reality, my mourning – here and now.

By writing this book, I am reminded of her children's participation. In my grief, I had simply forgotten what they had done. Although the year has gone by quickly, we covered a lot of ground and it was one of discovery and one of love.

I continue to be reminded that my attitude and need for control and perfection are my choices. I also realize I need to move on. Letting go does not mean we love her less.

My hope is that this book will bring closure, an appreciation for our love and innocence, and an understanding that death is part of life … part of living. Sharing my experience is my gift to my family, to my sister, and to me. It is my gift to you and to others who may be struggling in the same way.

It could be anyone's journey, but it's not … it's ours.

THE FIVE STAGES OF DEATH

Per Dr. Elisabeth Kübler-Ross
On Death and Dying

Shock

Denial

Anger

Bargaining

Acceptance

THE FIVE STAGES OF FAMILY GRIEF

Per Barbara Okun, Ph.D. and Joseph Nowinski, Ph.D.
Saying Goodbye: A Guide to Coping with a Loved One's Terminal Illness

Crisis

Unity

Upheaval

Resolution

Renewal

WAS HE TALKING TO ME?

"I have a secret," and she smiles. I lean forward in my chair to hear the news. "But, you can't tell." She goes on, "Lisa is pregnant. She used a home pregnancy test this morning. It revealed a slight pink line. She's waiting for the results of her blood test. She should know tomorrow."

My sister Carmen is sitting on her hospital bed; her body slightly leaning forward to facilitate her breathing – her usual posture. Arms at her sides, her hands are clinging to the mattress supporting her body weight. The sagging hospital gown is barely covering her shoulders; her thin legs are dangling, exposed; her feet are bare. Skin and bones, she looks so frail.

This is her first week in the hospital and the first week of knowing she has lung cancer. Therefore, we are both excited at the news of a grandchild – a sign of hope amid a week of emotional turmoil.

"OK. I won't tell but I'll call Mom so she can pray for Lisa tonight. This would be wonderful, you could share her pregnancy with her."

"It is a beautiful gift," and she smiles again.

This is the first time we are alone since the events of the past week began to unfold. A tear flows down her cheek then a second. She reaches for the box of Kleenex. I sit next to her on the bed holding her in my arms – trying to comfort her, afraid to break her. She wipes her eyes and then her nose. Her head tilted forward, looking down, she shares, "I don't want to bring you sorrow, to any of you. I don't want to hurt you."

She's concerned with us at a time like this? She knows how we feel; she's experienced it with Dad. What about her own feelings? Is this not a good time to be self-centred? I am at a loss for words.

It's too soon to tell her I'll miss her. Another day I'll tell her I'm sorry she has to live through this. Today, I'll tell her I love her.

Carmen is eight years my senior. As children we were not close. The Miller family dynamics at the time did not foster a warm, cozy, loving environment and we lived apart for many years during our childhood. We became close friends as young adults once I moved back to Ottawa.

"Bosom sisters" as Carmen used to say. A term she borrowed from Lucy Maud Montgomery in her favorite television series *Anne of Green Gables*.

Together we remain strong. I am rational and caring but not emotional in her presence. I do my best to envisage her needs and give her my support. I may not cry when we are together but I sob when we are not. So much so at times I think I'm falling apart.

Carmen wants us to pray so her daughter does not have another miscarriage. This pregnancy has more significance than it would otherwise have. It thrusts life into the focal point when death hovers stealthily like a vulture, a hungry predator continuously soaring without flapping its wings.

My sister needs this. She needs to know life continues. She needs something normal in her life, something to celebrate. She needs to escape reality.

It's been a while since I called on Him. I found myself still begging as I awaken the next morning. The results are in, it's confirmed, but her hormone levels are low. A few more blood tests are required. We should be able to announce the pregnancy shortly.

Rehydrated and with her pneumonia treated, Carmen is discharged from the hospital. Having experienced a temporary state of shock, she returns home a different woman, one whose life has changed forever, altered by terminal cancer.

Carmen's strength of character had diminished over the last few years. That said, she conveyed great wisdom and serenity from the very beginning in her approach and attitude towards death. Since that time, she had been preparing herself and her loved ones for her departure.

We exchange emails that week between my visits to her apartment.

> **September 27, 2011**
> **To Carmen – Subject: I have a secret**
> I love you very much. I am happy to see you back home and I'm so excited for you. You will be a grandmother! :) C U soon! Your bosom sister, Nicole
>
> **To Nicole** –I know some days will be hard but I am so happy you are my bosom and that we are a close family. Love you very

much and appreciate everything you are doing. Hum … wonder if you could be the godmother (with Martin as the godfather) and also the grandmother. I guess God is giving me one wish. Can't wait. Love you sis. Carmen

September 28, 2011
To Carmen – Subject: Grandmother
Nonna is the Italian word for grandmother. *Nonnina* is a term of endearment meaning "little grandmother". Occasionally, *nonnina* will be shortened to *nonni*, but *nonni* is also the word for grandparents plural. Nicole

September 29, 2011
To Nicole – I kind of like Nonna so Nonna it is. So remember we will both be called Nonna. Thank you for everything – being a friend, a sister and my bosom. Love you. Carmen

Our close-knit family is vital to Carmen's survival and to us all in coping with this awful fatal disease. My sister accepts that she will not be alive to see her grandchild grow up. She wants me to replace her as the grandmother when the time comes. In the meantime, she is searching for a name. She is not fond of "Mammy" or "Grand-maman" – she prefers a name unique to her. A special name her grandchild can call her.

Our conversations are soon interrupted when my sister's dream is shattered. Lisa has another miscarriage. She calls her mother sobbing. Carmen is devastated. How can this happen?

"HE can't do this. HE can't take my life and not give her a baby. HE can't do this." My sister is angry yet she remains at her daughter's side giving her the support she needs. Her children remain her priority.

"Everything happens for a reason." Words not to be shared with one who has been given a terminal diagnosis.

★ ★ ★

I never saw it coming. A week earlier, on Sunday September 18, 2011, I returned home from a golf weekend with my girlfriends. I called Carmen, as I usually do, when I return home from a trip. We had not spoken for a few days. I leave a message on her voice mail. I had no idea she was in the hospital, that she was ill. No one told me.

Her daughter Lisa returns my call shortly afterwards. She was at her mother's picking up a few items to bring to the hospital and heard my message. She explains that Carmen had dialed 911 the night before, due to severe diarrhea and vomiting. She was taken to the nearest hospital in her French community of Gatineau, Quebec. Once in emergency, she was isolated and placed in quarantine.

Carmen did not want her children to tell anyone. She did not want to bother anyone. She did not want us to worry. This was not the first time she made such a request. She had done the same back in 2007 when she had a collapsed lung the weekend Ron died (Ron was one of her ex-husbands and her children's biological father). That weekend I scolded my sister. My true ex-smoker attitude was at its best. "How can you continue to smoke? You have emphysema, just like Dad, are you waiting to have cancer before quitting? You know how difficult it was for us when Dad passed away, how can you do this to your children?" She quit smoking that day.

★ ★ ★

September 18, 2011
I wait for news. I'm not sure if we can visit her while she is in quarantine.

Later I am told that Carmen has pneumonia. The emergency physician is concerned there could be something more and requested additional tests. She is to remain in quarantine for a few days until a bed can be assigned to her.

I remember my younger sister Joanne telling me, "It can be serious. People can die of pneumonia. I know of a few." Little did we realize we would be adding one more name to the list.

Later that Sunday, Carmen's son Martin announces the shocking news, regardless of his mother asking him not to. He phones me on his way home from the hospital. His voice is calm. He proceeds to tell me, "My mom has cancer."

The shocking news sends an immediate bolt of lightning through my entire body. As he hears his own voice, he begins to cry. It brought me back to over a decade ago when Dad was diagnosed with lung cancer.

Concerned about Martin crying and driving at the same time, I order him to park his van or hang up, get a hold of himself and call me when he gets home.

In my panic, I run outside looking for Roger. I find him in the front yard dressed in his maintenance clothes: grass stained jeans, an old shirt and a straw hat to protect him from the sun. With the "whipper snipper" in hand, he is trimming the lawn around the flowerbeds. I startle him when I tap his shoulder from behind. His look is strange. Mine, I'm sure, reflects my state of mind. He removes one ear muff to listen to my cries. His strange look quickly turns to one of fright once I give him the news. "What type of cancer?" I run back into the house and phone Martin: it is lung cancer. It can't be, I thought, it just can't be. My sister can't have lung cancer.

It's not uncommon for cancer patients to keep their diagnosis private. They don't want to be treated differently. They are in shock: they are traumatized.

Disregarding the fact that visiting hours are coming to an end, Roger and I leave for the hospital. I insist on driving. I know Roger will respect the speed limit and drive slower than me, but I want to get there fast. I want to be with my sister.

En route I hear Roger say, "Go. Hurry. Drive faster!" I look down at the speedometer. To my surprise, I'm actually driving 20 km below the speed limit; I'm doing 40 km in a 60 zone when my norm is usually 80. My world is unfolding in slow motion – the movie reel doesn't want to turn any faster. What's going on? This can't be. This isn't happening.

We walk into the quarantine area as if we belong. No questions asked by hospital personnel. We spot Carmen through the glass wall of her isolation cubicle.

Although we spoke often on the phone, we had not seen each other for weeks. I knew my sister was tired, stressed and somewhat depressed. In late August, her family physician had given her a medical leave for three months. He thought she was suffering from depression as a result of her separation from George and the lawsuit with the housing corporation. Earlier that afternoon, Lisa and I were actually sharing how we could help and where to solicit counselling. We were not prepared for what was coming.

I peek through the glass wall. Carmen is lying in bed. She turns to look at the sound of the door opening. She is pleasantly surprised to see us. We share a hug and kiss. Roger does the same. My sister looks frail and much older than her 59 years. She reminds me of Dad when he was hospitalized. She too has lost so much weight, and quickly. Down to 96 lbs, she lost a total of 30 in the last few months.

How did this happen? This is a nightmare. This is surreal. Our lives have changed in a matter of seconds.

We don't say much. We don't need to. Eventually she shares, "Well, I did smoke. You just never think it's going to happen to you."

"No one deserves cancer regardless of whether they were a smoker or not!" was my response.

She remains strong and calm. She informs us the cancer is in both lungs. I feel numb.

I proceed by asking if she had submitted her notice of retirement and resignation to her employer as planned. She did not. "Thank God," I say. Thank God for her procrastination. This means she continues to be eligible for health benefits when she will need them the most.

Roger and I leave the hospital with a profound sadness. I let him drive. I phone my family en route home. I soon change my cell phone plan to unlimited long distance calls and texting. We are a close family and will become much closer. We will be in contact almost daily.

The next morning, Joanne and I head to the hospital. Joanne prefers to visit Carmen together with me, afraid if she went alone that she would cry and not be much support to our sister. Joanne, the youngest of the six siblings, had accompanied Dad for his initial visit to the oncologist. When the latter delivered the deadly news, Dad found himself comforting Joanne instead of vice versa. She thought we would be stronger if we stood together.

As I'm driving to the hospital Lisa phones me on my cell – she is crying. It becomes apparent Martin and Lisa are lost souls. When Dad was sick, we had Mom to guide us. Carmen's children have us. We agree to meet them after our visit with their mother.

Lisa continues by asking us what she should say to people who are calling. Carmen had asked her children not to disclose she has cancer. They feel awkward not being able to share this with neighbours and friends, particularly George. Everyone is concerned; all are inquiring about her health. I plan to discuss it with Carmen and will have an answer for Lisa this afternoon.

Carmen and George's relationship ended one year before her diagnosis; the reason is irrelevant. They had not spoken since. Their relationship has been an intermittent one for the past 40 years, like Elizabeth Taylor and Richard Burton.

Living in the adjacent apartment building, George saw the ambulance arrive earlier that week. He quickly ran to the paramedics as they were helping Carmen enter the ambulance. The Ottawa ambulance was redirected to Gatineau to respond to my sister's call. An intercity, interprovincial agreement allows for such service to counter the shortage of ambulances in Gatineau. The Ottawa paramedics did not speak French and were not familiar with the location of the hospital. George gave them directions. He offered to take his car so they might follow him. They refused. Too weak and confused to think of asking to lie on the stretcher, Carmen followed directives and sat on the bench next to the paramedic. She declined George's offer to accompany her to the hospital. Anxious and concerned he pled, "You must let your children know. Do you want me to phone them?" And so he did.

★ ★ ★

Joanne and I arrive at the hospital. I'm surprised to see Carmen's co-worker in the quarantine room. I was expecting us to be alone. I learn later that Julie is a close friend of hers. She stays a while and leaves. Once the sisters are alone, I mention to Carmen that we will be meeting with her children to help them deal with this. I also suggest that they be able to share with people that she has cancer. George is calling, co-workers and neighbours are calling – they are all worried. The children are in a difficult situation. She agrees. She adds, "If George wants to come and visit, he can."

Joanne and I make it to Lisa's later that morning. When Martin arrives, brother and sister hug for a while. It's nice to see they are close. We have lunch but we are not hungry.

We reminisce and share with them our experience with Dad and his cancer and what they can expect. I finish by saying how lucky I was to have shared my father's journey with him. "It was one of the most enriching experiences in my life." I add, "Don't miss this opportunity with your mom."

"We need to prepare ourselves mentally for the worst." I continue, "We don't know if your mother's cancer is terminal but we do know it's in both lungs. She also has emphysema. Is the cancer in the healthy portion of her lungs or the dead tissue? We don't know. Either way it does not look promising."

Lisa is sitting at the end of the kitchen table sobbing, "I don't know what to say to her when I see her." We encourage them to be open with their mother, to share their feelings.

"I remember telling my dad I was going to miss him; that I felt like he was going on a trip, an adventure somewhere and that we would see each other later. I remember telling him I love him." I add, "You know, this is also new for your mom. This time, she's the one with cancer. We are all on a learning curve. The best thing we can do is to be open about our feelings."

★ ★ ★

The family crisis had already begun. It seems to happen naturally when a loved one is diagnosed with cancer. The many calls, all justified, from family members looking for answers and looking for comfort. The unknown, the panic, the anxiety become a common, almost synchronized reaction. We want to be by her side. We don't know what to do. One of us has lung cancer. It's frightening.

As soon as George heard the news, he was quickly at my sister's side and remained with her until her passing 12 months later. We can't say enough about his generosity and his love for my sister.

Later that week Carmen is assigned a hospital room. She can now receive phone calls, to the dismay of her roommate.

They continue with more tests, including a CT Scan and a bronchoscopy. George is with her throughout the week. Partial test results arrive at different times, delivered by different physicians and specialists.

The blow comes on Friday, September 23, 2011. A stranger walks into the room. He doesn't bother to introduce himself. His attire implies a health care worker. He proceeds by delivering the drastic news to Carmen and George.

Carmen is in shock, George even more so. She is told she has cancer in both lungs. Her cancer is already at stage IV. It is inoperable and terminal. Treatments will not prolong her life or cure her cancer. The prognosis is 12-18 months. It is delivered in a cold, factual and seemingly detached uncaring manner.

She remains calm through one of the most traumatic moments one can live – knowing your mortality is here and now. I can't imagine receiving such news.

Death is inevitable. We all know we will die; however, we don't expect it in the near future. We assume it will be much later when we are older, when our life has been fulfilled.

George brings himself to speak. His only question, "Can we do a transplant? Can I give her one of my lungs?"

George was Carmen's first fiancé. I was ten years old at the time. He was my hero back then. He still is.

"She would not survive an operation. She has emphysema and her lungs are too weak." The stranger turns to look at Carmen, "An appointment will be scheduled with an oncologist to determine your treatments, your chemotherapy. Again, it won't cure your cancer or prolong your life; it will only improve your quality of life."

The stranger, dressed in a clinical white coat, leaves the room. They never knew his name. They assume he's a physician. He came and went like a cold gust of wind. One would think delivering such news is an art. Compassion and empathy are obviously not mastered by all physicians. Should they be? Is it not part of patient care? Is it because physicians need to detach themselves? Having a better appreciation of what their patients and families go through would better serve their patients and themselves. Guiding a patient at end-of-life can be enriching to physicians if they choose. If they prefer not to, then why not delegate the task to other members of the health care team, or better yet, work as a team with members who are better qualified in this area and have a more humane approach.

The stranger leaves my sister thinking, "Was he talking to me?"

Carmen refrains from sharing the news until the timing is right. She schedules a meeting with her children for the next morning. She wants to speak with them together. They know she received word from the physician. They sense bad news. Carmen rehearsed her speech many times. The three will cry together.

That Friday night, my sister Denise arrives for the weekend. She lives in the village of Saint-Sauveur, Quebec. A popular ski destination located in the Laurentian Mountains, a two-hour drive from Ottawa.

I'm attending a motorcycle rider training course for the next two days. During that time my two older sisters spend time together. They too are close. Denise is the eldest of the six siblings. Two years older than Carmen.

Saturday night, Denise shares with me the results of Carmen's latest tests, regardless of Carmen's wishes to wait until my rider training course and practical test are over. "Carmen's cancer is at stage IV. Both lungs and the liver are affected. The prognosis is she has 12 to 18 months to live."

Sitting at home in my library, glass of wine in hand, we cry again.

Sunday morning I have more driving lessons. My practical test is scheduled for the afternoon. I phone Joanne and Denise during the morning break – it hit me when speaking with Joanne. They had just announced the latest news to our brother David and to Mom. I begin sobbing on the telephone. "Get a hold of yourself," says Joanne. A common response lately.

Although I walk away, another student overhears my conversation. I debate if I should complete or quit the course. I'm more than half way through; if I quit now I will have to redo the course in its entirety. My three sisters are together. There is nothing more I can do.

I continue the day in tears; my eyes are like a leaking faucet. Everyone avoids me once they know what's happening. My concentration is low and I can't seem to grasp the instructions. I hear them, I understand, but strangely enough I can't follow through. I can't execute. I barely pass my practical test. I ask for the necessary paperwork and decline to do the honorary drive around the campus as a group. I want out, I need to leave.

Most of the instructors are smokers. I refrain from sharing my thoughts as the coordinator hands me my papers. I so want to tell him, "If you love your six-year-old daughter you would quit smoking." But I do not. I thank him and leave. He probably would have thought – *it won't happen to me.* Just like a sexually-active teenager without birth control.

"You must be fully alert when driving a motorcycle. The impact of your mental state is crucial to your survival." A tip shared by an instructor and one I have not forgotten; one which explains why I could not execute the tasks.

The next day I'm at Chapters Indigo. I need the self-help section and more. How do we deal with this? How can I help my sister? What do we do?

The best book on the shelf is *Help me live – 20 things people with cancer want you to know.*

Our journey is underway.

ENOUGH WITH THE REINFORCEMENT

Two rings indicate a long distance phone call. It's Roger – they killed a buck. He shares his first bow hunting experience. He's on his way home. He's been gone for more than a week. He never asked how Carmen was nor did I bring it up. I return to my book *Help me live* … the first chapter is entitled "*It's okay to say or do the wrong thing.*" I realize this is foreign to him.

By the time Carmen returns home from the hospital, she has been out of the office for over a month. After communicating with her employer, she learns all her sick days and holidays have been used. In effect, beginning early October, she is no longer on the payroll and therefore not eligible for health benefits. She would have to cover both the employer and employee premiums for coverage. Long-term disability is possible only after three months. They do not offer short-term disability. She has no revenue coming in. What a mega pickle.

Carmen has several discussions with her manager Greg. He informs her that an employee has to be on the payroll ten days in a month to be eligible for health benefits. He suggests she opt for the possibility of purchasing the four days she has missing. She agrees and her benefits continue for the month of October.

Greg is attending a conference at the Fairmont Chateau Laurier Hotel in downtown Ottawa. He agrees to meet me in the spacious lobby with its impressive marble floors and exquisite furnishings. I sit next to the limestone fireplace and admire the massive log ceiling and wide moldings while I wait. I don't know who to look for.

I approach a man holding a briefcase, "Are you here to meet Nicole?" I ask.

"No, I'm not."

I return to my seat. I wonder how call girls do it. I continue observing the traffic. A bald man arrives, sits on a leather bench and scans the room. He's holding a brown legal size envelope. It must be him. I walk across the room.

"Are you Greg?"

His smile confirms he is.

We introduce ourselves. Sitting next to him, I note the lingering smell of nicotine on his clothes. He hands me the envelope containing insurance forms and other documentation. He briefly explains what's required. I take in the instructions with hesitance. I'm somewhat doubtful of his approach given the reputation of insurance companies.

Discreetly chewing gum, he informs me he is a cancer survivor. He is genuine when he shares his concerns for my sister's welfare, "I've worked with Carmen for 21 years; I've known her longer than any of my wives!"

I return to my sister with the documentation. I don't impose; I leave her in control of her personal affairs. I respect her autonomy and I am sensitive to her physical and mental state. I wait until she is ready for my help.

★ ★ ★

The trial is in a few days. I contact my sister's lawyer. The date needs to be rescheduled given her condition. She will never be physically or psychologically able to attend. Her lawyer is disappointed to hear of Carmen's health. She remains astounded that this group continues to pursue the lawsuit against my sister. It's unjustified, a waste of time, energy and money for everyone. The only thing her lawyer can do is keep deferring the date.

The lawsuit is one of malice and orchestrated by a few to get back at my sister for her years on the board of the cooperative where she resides. Regardless of her innocence, being sued was extremely stressful for my sister. It is for anyone. I have no doubt that it affected her overall health.

★ ★ ★

Sharing news among family members brings on additional fatigue. One night can represent six or seven telephone calls if not more, all with the same message. It becomes easier to keep them informed through emails. I include the immediate family except for Carmen. A total of 20 members receive my emails. My sister is aware of my correspondence but I don't add her to my list, not yet.

September 27, 2011
Hello everyone,
It's been quite the emotional week. Good news – Carmen is going home today. She will be meeting her oncologist October 20th, at which time they will decide on her chemotherapy. I take it he will have a better idea of how much time she has based on the results of her biopsy.

She is doing well but of course this is a hard pill to swallow. She is truly taking it one day at a time and I guess we need to do the same (we just need to figure out how to block those tear ducts!). Now that she will be back home and feeling better she will have access to her email. A few words of encouragement and news of yourselves, what you are up to … would change her thoughts. I probably don't need to say it but I know she will be pleased to hear from you.

Martin and Lisa, we think of your mother and we think of you. I don't believe you will need to ask for help but if ever we miss out on anything, please do not hesitate to ask – otherwise we will be hurt. We love you very much. We are very lucky to have each other. Remember … we are family … :)

If any of you want to come for a visit – our doors are open. Please feel free; anytime. A big hug to all of you. Nicole

P.S. I guess this really brings it home. Life is precious – don't sweat the small stuff.

September 29, 2011
Hello again,
Carmen, George and I have been spending the last few days together. We are like the three musketeers. We have a date next week to drive in Gatineau Park to see the fall colours.

Carmen's spirits are good. When she's down, she gives herself a few minutes to cry and then she moves on. She now weighs 104 pounds. The jujubes, chips, chocolate bars don't seem to work on her but they do on my waistline. Thanks George!

Carmen needs to rebuild her strength. Just walking from the entrance of the hospital to the oncology department was too much for her today. No treatments yet, we simply dropped off insurance forms for her oncologist to sign. The visit gave Carmen a chance to speak to other patients about their chemo experience. Scary!

She's happy to be back home. And happy we are a close family ... so am I.

Hugs to all. Nicole

★ ★ ★

Carmen prefers to remain in her apartment by herself. George stayed with her for the first few nights and then returned to his own apartment. He lives close by. He tucks her in at night and is there with her breakfast in the morning. He prepares her lunch. He bathes her. He cleans her apartment. He does so much. He has taken the role of primary caregiver. I'm second in command. Everyone else comes and goes.

Martin walks into his mother's apartment with a cup of Tim Hortons coffee in hand and a bag in the other. He's gained weight this past year. Probably a result of his stressful business and personal relationships, but you would never know it. He always greets you with a smile. He greets everyone with a smile, just like his uncle David.

"Hey Mom, I received the two keyless locks. I'll install them for you today." He hands her the bag. She smiles as she takes out the muffin, a fruit explosion. Carmen is pleased with the keyless locks. She provides the combination to family and close friends. This makes it easier for her. She no longer needs to get up to unlock the door for us. We respect her privacy. We phone ahead, we don't drop in unexpectedly.

I share my knowledge with my family, including Carmen. I know my bosom sister; I hope my emails will be helpful to her in understanding what she is living through. My summaries become our new channel for communication.

September 29, 2011
Hello again,
I've come across this book *Help me live – 20 things people with cancer want you to know*. The author, Lori Hope, is a cancer survivor who surveyed some 600 patients. The book is targeted not only at family and friends but also at cancer survivors, hence my email to the entire family; including Carmen. My thought was to share with you a synopsis of every chapter as I go through the book. It may be helpful to us in this journey.

Help me live: Chapter 1 – "It's okay to say or do the wrong thing."

- Sometimes we are afraid of saying the wrong thing. Keep it simple. Be honest – it shows you care.
- Nobody's perfect. If you say the wrong thing, apologize – it's OK. People will forgive you.
- At times we feel uncomfortable and awkward. We think we should provide wise and helpful words. Perhaps the most important thing we can give each other is our attention. A loving silence can have more power and connection than well-intentioned words.
- "I don't know what to say," are words that never fail.
- Sometimes our expectations of loved ones are too high. Somehow we feel they should know what to say or do. Know that we are trying to understand how the other feels.
- We may feel guilt or shame and are focusing on ourselves rather than the person we want to help.
- You don't need to talk all the time. At times calm and quiet is what is needed.

- Don't be fearful. Sometimes we are so guarded and frightened that we stay away from the people who need us more than anything.
- Treat the person like a family member and not a cancer patient.
- Doing nothing or holding back may be worse than doing too much or saying the wrong thing.
- If you have an impulse to hug someone – obey.
- It's OK to cry.
- Most newly diagnosed patients prefer to talk about their own experience than those of others.
- Practice self-compassion and forgiveness.
- Errors are understandable and forgivable.

Sometimes doing the wrong thing turns out to be a gift for many others. One woman, Susan Halpern, neglected to visit a sick neighbour. Her regrets led to writing the book *The Etiquette of Illness – a resource book for caregivers.* Another woman, Debbie Sardone, who owned a house cleaning service turned down a woman with cancer who could not afford her. She later founded "Cleaning for a Reason," a non-profit that helps provide free house cleanings for people undergoing cancer treatment. Lori Hope, the author of *Help me live*, could not have supported her mother better. Her book is helping us today.

"To avoid situations in which you might make mistakes may be the biggest mistakes of all."[5]

I hope this was of interest. Hug someone today. Nicole XO

Carmen's reply
Thank you Nicole. Hi everybody, everything is fine. I am taking it one day at a time and allowed to cry five minutes a day, not more. Very thankful God gave me such a loving family. Love you all. Carmen

---

[5] Peter McWilliams

Lisa and her husband James cuddle together on the couch. James reads every line of my email aloud. They share thoughts on the various points. I am pleased my efforts are helpful. We all want to learn. I am not alone in supporting my sister.

> **September 30, 2011** Carmen sends Denise and me an email. She begins to share her thoughts and her feelings.
>
> Hi everybody,
> As you know, I am allowed to cry only five minutes a day but I can't for two more days because I used them yesterday. So I thought I would share with you what goes through my brain when I wake up in the morning (usually my crying time). Today I was thinking the hardest part is to say goodbye when the time comes, but I am so grateful I have a loving family and I love you all so much. I don't think I am scared of dying; I did not do anything bad. I hope God will let me in. Anyway, if some of you don't want me to send you what I think, let me know. I will not be mad or offended. And no, I did not cry; still two days to go.
> Love you, Carmen
>
> **My reply**
> Carmen, that was beautiful. Maybe we should also restrict ourselves to five minutes a day. I've cc'd the entire family so they too can cry! We love you and we will miss you.
> Your bosom sister, Nicole

Eventually, Carmen feels smothered. She is suffocating with our presence, our help, our advice, our phone calls ... at times she finds herself counselling family and friends.

"I should not have told anyone," she says.

I realize it's too much reinforcement at once. Not uncommon during a family crisis. We are at her side, jumping at every command, reorganizing her life and ours. We buy her groceries, cook her meals, do her errands, rearrange her furniture, clean her apartment and accompany her to medical appointments. Are we giving her too much support? Are we imposing our love? We don't believe it's too much fuss. We want her to be comfortable. We don't want her to suffer. We don't know what else to do.

Carmen has mixed feelings. Every day is different. Sometimes she feels angry yet she wants our support. At times she wants her space yet she needs our love. She wants her autonomy but she is physically unable to do so many things one takes for granted. She does not have the energy or the strength. She often voices, "I am a prisoner of my body."

October 2, 2011
Hello everyone,
You will notice Julie's name in the family group listing. She's one of Carmen's closest friends and our newly adopted sister. You probably met Julie at Lisa's wedding. She makes great tasting fudge. She finds these summaries beneficial so I included her in my mailings.

Here's a synopsis of…

Help me live: Chapter 2 – "I need to know you're here for me, but if you can't be, you can still show you care."

- All of us want to believe that our friends and family will be there when we need them most.
- Our deepest fear is that they will not be.
- The reality is some people will be and others will not.
- Not everyone can deal with life threatening situations. Some can't deal with the disease. Being sick scares us all. Don't stay away because of it. You can be there without talking about it.
- The reason some people are not there for their loved ones, is that they just don't know what to do. Then why not ask?
- Some are unable to be there – they just aren't psychologically able to do it. It is difficult. Don't be afraid to talk about it. Share your thoughts/concerns. (Personally, I physically feel it when I see a sore; it can range from a sick feeling in my stomach to diarrhea and vomiting. I experienced the latter after looking at Patrick's eye operation. On the other hand, Carmen loves to show her wounds – and usually more than once. So what a pair we will make!)
- Cancer is not contagious.

- Be there without being there. Being there can be face-to-face, voice-to-voice … it can be a brief note, a voicemail, a text, an email, a special gesture. It can mean the world to someone with cancer. What matters is that they know you care, that they matter to you.
- Neglect is just as painful as harsh judgment words.
- "I'm here whenever you need me," are the words one loves to hear.
- The only things for sure in life are death and taxes … and with taxes we know when they will occur.

What I love about this book is that it helps us, as a family, to better communicate and be open. It helps me understand what people with cancer and their loved ones go through. It helps me be there.

I love you all. Let's give each other another hug. See you soon. Nicole

Carmen's reply
Really good summary. I love you all and give you a big hug everyone. Thanks again. Nicole, I guess I am keeping you very busy in your retirement.

Carmen's experiences and feelings are no different than those identified in my summaries. It is evident, based on my discussions with her and on her outlook, that the summaries are insightful. They serve as a guide to help us understand, forgive and avoid being judgmental with family, friends and strangers. Our communication improves. We gain a common language.

Jennifer, a cousin, phones Carmen. They used to be friends but have not spoken for over a decade. Jennifer had been disrespectful with our mother and Carmen disassociated herself from her as a result.

Jennifer is calling, asking for forgiveness. Carmen is not upset with her. Whatever happened was a long time ago, she does not want to waste her energy on something so trivial. She does not hold a grudge. She does not have time. She shares with our cousin that she prefers no visitors at this time. She is too tired, too weak and ill, "Maybe you can visit me later Jennifer, when I feel better."

★ ★ ★

I wonder if the human body prepares for death physically and psychologically. Similarities between Dad and Carmen are evident – the physical traits, postures and mannerisms. The same type of cancer brings on similar pain.

When my father was diagnosed with terminal lung cancer, he often appeared pensive or in a daze. So does Carmen. "Remember when we wondered what Dad was thinking of? And he would say nothing." She adds, "It's nothing. Often I think of nothing."

This is Carmen's journey. We witness a gradual transformation as she prepares to leave this world. Every night she thanks God for the day He has given her and every morning she wakes she thanks Him for giving her another day. She feels blessed that she has the opportunity to say goodbye to those she loves and is able to spend precious moments with them knowing it won't last forever.

"I would much rather die of cancer than a heart attack. This way I have a chance to say goodbye." This is Carmen's view. My brother David has a different opinion. Having experienced a heart attack nine months earlier at the age of 55, his thought is, "I would rather die of a heart attack and go quickly than to see and feel my body deteriorate."

As a family we remain open about Carmen's cancer, her outlook and her journey. My expectations are based on my experience. I read on the subject, I think I'm well versed. I approach this with a mission – my goal is to help my sister. It's all about her. Or is it?

Mourning someone who is living brings on a broad range of emotions, sometimes with complexity; sometimes they're uncharacteristic. You manage your feelings and others do the same. Everyone's emotions can easily collide with one another. There is no room for judgment. The imminent loss is stressful for everyone including Carmen. This becomes our new "normal".

★ ★ ★

All medical appointments and exams are demanding physically and psychologically. My sister's calendar is full. It takes her days to recuperate, especially if they inject contrast material into her body. She now has a PICC line inserted in her left arm (a form of intravenous access, the PICC line will be used for drawing blood samples, chemotherapy, antibiotics and pain medication). It will be cleaned and flushed with saline by a nurse once a week. Eventually it gets to be too much for my sister to make it to the clinic. The nurse is asked to come to her apartment instead.

"When do you begin your chemo?" the nurse asks.

"I don't know. I'm meeting Dr. Jones for the first time on October 20th. He's my oncologist."

"He's one physician who always orders PICC lines too early. Sometimes a patient has it months before their treatment." The nurse continues, "It's additional work for us."

Carmen has been living in fear for weeks. She's terrified of her upcoming appointment with her oncologist. Terrified of more bad news. Terrified of the unknown.

"Helloooooooooooooooooooooo?" A typical early morning email from Carmen. If we were up, she was ready to talk.

> **October 3, 2011 to Denise and me**
> Good morning,
> Well, I had a tough night last night. I tried to sleep with Aunt Lora's rosary between my breasts but they are too small and saggy so the rosary kept falling. Thought of Louise, who I have to write to. We have been friends since 1974. She is very special so I want to be the one to tell her. Nicole, I don't know if you want to come on the 20th. Do not want to impose it on you but you are welcome. Feel free to decide, I will not be hurt by your decision. Talk to you later. Love you. Carmen
>
> **My reply**
> I've been thinking of Louise. I know it's hard for you to tell her. She's probably your longest, closest friend. She'll simply send more love your way. Shit, now I'm crying! I did not tell you but as for the 20th I plan to meet you at the entrance of the hospital and give you a great big hug before you go in. I think it's best if you see the oncologist with George and the kids otherwise the doctor will feel like you are coming in with an army. I will be there when you come out. :)

With the size of beads on that rosary no wonder you didn't sleep!

October 3, 2011
Hello everyone,
Carmen is doing well however, she's very tired from the weekend. Maybe too many calls … maybe too many guests … maybe too many activities. That's what happens when too many of us care. I guess we'll have to limit her activities to one dance a day.

Here's a summary of …

Help me live: Chapter 3 – "I like to hear success stories; not horror stories."

- Many people want to make it seem like they can relate to what you are going through and tell you about people they know who had cancer. It's not comforting.
- Stories can be terrifying.
- There is absolutely no way that a person who has not had cancer can fully understand the feeling of absolute vulnerability and terrorizing fear that occurs when you hear the diagnosis of cancer.
- Some people need to share their personal stories because they are still grieving. They don't realize at that moment that their stories are horror stories. We have to have a special tolerance and understanding of anyone who has suffered a loss. Telling their story is their survival – their healing.
- Survivors need and love success stories. The circumstances must at least match those of the survivor, e.g., similar age, equal or more advanced stage of the same cancer.
- Sometimes people just can't help stuffing their foot in their mouth. I say go back to Chapter One!
- Be mindful – it may take several success stories to mitigate the impact of one horror story.

Collect hopeful tales and keep them closely guarded in your heart.

Knowing how to compassionately treat someone who has been traumatized comes more naturally to one who can put himself in another's shoes.

Have a great day. Love, Nicole XO

Carmen's reply
Well, this is my five-minute crying time. You are doing an excellent job. I guess I am keeping a few people up.

October 4, 2011
Hello again,
It can make a world of difference when you meet a health care provider who is compassionate, knowledgeable and caring. Hopefully, Carmen will meet this nurse again ... and again. I did not know this but the PICC line (set up in prep for chemo) is a long tube inserted in her upper left arm, which goes to her heart. Of course, Carmen could not wait to share all details with me.

No need to worry if you have a cold at one of our gatherings, Carmen now has a box of face masks for protection.

Help me live: Chapter 5 – "I need you to listen to me and let me cry."

- Don't be uncomfortable with silence. Sometimes it's the best answer.
- Just listen. Try to understand. Keep your eyes and ears open and your mouth shut.
- When someone verbalizes their fears, don't minimize it or trivialize it. Be supportive.
- Support groups provide a medium for sharing without being concerned about worrying loved ones.
- Be present emotionally. Open your heart.
- Part of the skill of listening is to acknowledge the pain, absorb it and very important, to let it go.
- Allow one to share their feelings. You don't need to fix it. You don't need to know the answers.

- "Tell me how you are doing," helps to bring something out of the person.
- Hold hands.
- Being diagnosed with cancer is a surreal experience. Telling your story makes it real. It is important to talk about it – over and over again. It's sometimes painful but therapeutic.
- It's OK to talk about it and it's OK to cry. It helps us get through the process.

Emotional tears contain two kinds of stress hormones and as they leave the body through the eyes, they create a calming effect (plus give you really puffy eyes and a red nose!). See you soon.
Nicole XO

October 5, 2011
Hi everyone,
Sometimes when Carmen thinks of her initial meeting with the physician – she wonders, "Was he talking to me?"

Help me live: Chapter 4 – "I am terrified and need to know you'll forgive me if I snap at you or bite your head off."

- The first emotion most people diagnosed with cancer experience is terror – not only of death and difficult treatment but of being abandoned because they feel so angry, confused and out of control. They may say or do things out of character that are sometimes hurtful.
- Many who have had cancer experience frequent and intense emotional mood swings. They may react one way one day, and may react differently to the same words or actions the next day.
- Personalities can jump from Jekyll to Hyde in seconds (not to be confused with PMS or pre-menopause!). Often, people with cancer snap and blow up without knowing why. They may be transferring their anger about cancer to whoever happens to be close by at the time.
- Don't take what is said personally. Don't bitch back unless it's really out of hand.

- Forgive.
- Be patient when loved ones shut you out. Moods can change rapidly because of the disease and/or treatments. Don't give up on them.
- Loaded words can make you snap. Don't assume you know where one is at on any given day.
- Remission is not a comforting word – cure or cancer free sounds much better.
- It's OK to express our fears. Truly listen.

They say of the five senses, deprivation of touch is the most severe. A sincere hug allows us to feel cared about. Group hug folks. :) Nicole

From Jekyll to Hyde in seconds is no exaggeration. Ironically enough, the one who does the most for her is the one who is targeted. This is not unique to my sister; it is very common among critically ill patients and their caregivers. On many occasions Carmen is vicious with George. He is the target for most of her anger. The reasons vary … his presence; he is late; he and others do not understand what she is living; he does not read my summaries; he is in denial; the sound of the vacuum cleaner is too loud; he buys the wrong cereal; he buys too much or not enough; it's too healthy, etc. The good man that he is, he continues to do his best to care for her.

"I don't know how I would react if I was in her shoes," he tells me.

October 5, 2011
Me again,

Help me live: Chapter 6 – "Asking my permission can spare me pain."

Ask permission before:

- Heaping your troubles on someone who has cancer.
- Talking about your own fears (rely on other family and friends instead).
- Discussing treatment options.
- Preparing & delivering meals (sometimes the sight or smell of certain or all foods is unbearable during treatments). Great

if people put their names on the casseroles — easier to return the dishes.
- Sharing the news about someone's cancer (they may not want to discuss their illness with others).
- A visit. You do not want people coming by uninvited for many reasons. Even calling an hour ahead to check if the person is still up to it is appreciated.
- Bringing a pet.
- Sending articles/stories on cancer. Read them first to see if one with cancer would like such articles.

It just hit me — there are a few chapters in this book! Nicole

October 5, 2011
You are doing a great job. I noticed I am allowed only one activity a day because I get very tired. So sorry if sometimes I have to reschedule you but I would not be good company. I noticed also I am more alive in the morning; after 1 P.M. I have burnt all my energy. Love you guys. Carmen

October 6, 2011
Good morning everyone.
Today I was thinking it would be best if I store my car for the winter. George and others can give me lifts or I can take a taxi. I won't have the hassle of taking the car out for the cleaning crew when we have a snowstorm. With the treatments I doubt I will feel like driving. So that was my thought for today. Carmen

October 7, 2011
Just for the record, when it's my turn to give Carmen a bath, I'll walk in with rubber gloves (to the elbows) and a Carol Burnett mop. Please do not ask me who Carol Burnett is — that would really make me feel old!

Help me live: Chapter 7 – "I need to laugh – or just forget about cancer for a while."

- Sometimes people want a temporary pass from Cancerland. They need to laugh and laugh some more.
- Humour is a common coping mechanism.
- Laughter can make you feel less fearful and anxious.
- Some say comedy can cure.
- Complain daily but make an appointment to laugh everyday.
- Laugh out loud. It is contagious. Enroll in a laughter yoga session (let's try this when we next get together. I can already picture Carmen's face!).
- We can be in a bad mood; we can cry or feel sorry for ourselves. We choose the emotion that will serve us at that time.
- Tumor humour – not recommended.
- The best you can do as a caregiver is give space to really mourn and give space to really have fun.
- Laughter decreases your stress hormones.
- Offer the gift of laughter.

Don't lose your sense of humour. It's your most precious possession. Smile, Nicole XO

October 7, 2011
I don't know if George wants to give that spot away. He quite enjoys giving me a bath. Sometimes the water gets cold, takes him too long. Wonder why. Carmen

October 10, 2011
Had a great supper at Nicole's. Did not know my sister could cook. Her sugar pie was delicious. Well, today is really a shitty day. Been up since 4 and my eyes can't stop dripping. Don't know why and since I don't know why, my five minutes don't count. Oh, and Nicole gave me her leftovers; I think she gave me the whole bird. Thank God George has a great appetite. Carmen

Carmen attends to the necessary legal paperwork. She reviews her living will, power of attorney and testament. She selects the palliative care centre where she wants to spend her last days – one she supported for many years through the United Way. Once she is ready to make her funeral arrangements, I schedule an appointment with representatives of the funeral home and the cemetery. I am happy the three of us are doing this together. We are open and comfortable shopping and discussing the different options. Carmen smiles as she holds the urn like it was anything but. We laugh. I take a picture with my cellphone, "I look bruised" was her comment. My sister knows what she wants. No contracts are signed. We simply need to take action when the time comes. Later in the afternoon we select the picture to be placed next to the urn during the funeral. It's one taken nine months ago during a sisters' weekend at Denise's. Carmen is beautiful. The picture reveals no sign of illness.

I can't say I find it strange. I am better prepared this time. I felt awful when I accompanied my mother to purchase my father's casket. Walking into a room full of caskets to make a selection when my dad was in palliative care did not seem right to me. As she often did during that time, my mother pushed us to face reality. I felt even worse when she shared with Dad our selection and cost. I did not know he had asked her to do this. The doctor had told him the day before to get his things in order. The young physician held his hand, she hugged him and cried with him when she announced the cancer was progressing. He did not have much time left. My father was getting ready.

★ ★ ★

Carmen is still without revenue. We visit the local Service Canada Centre. It's important for her to look after her own affairs while she can. It gives her a sense of control plus she enjoys being a bitch on occasion – it's allowed – she has terminal cancer. She has only so many months to live and she does not hesitate to share it with faceless bureaucrats. It leaves them speechless. My sister can be quite direct at times. My husband is of the impression it's a family trait.

She walks in with an assertive attitude. It's physically apparent my sister is ill. She provides the clerk with a copy of her medical leave. She is told she must apply online for unemployment insurance benefits. It will take many weeks for the first payment to arrive, if she is eligible. They go on about their process. She doesn't hesitate to share her thoughts on their bureaucracy. In the meantime, I lend her money.

★ ★ ★

When a family is in crisis everyone is in shock. It creates a sense of panic and eventually brings unity among family members. That was our experience. Needless to say, it could be the opposite for any family. Depending on the personalities and their reaction to lingering family issues, the crisis could easily bring disunity.

As Carmen's illness progresses we are all at different phases in this growing experience. Some are in denial; others are moving forward – some maybe too fast, like me. I'm looking ahead. Being aware and responsible for her affairs, I'm stressed and very concerned for my sister's welfare.

Every aspect of Carmen's life seems complicated. Her current financial situation is bleak. She has no revenue, her medical coverage is uncertain, her insurance coverage is pending, she has financial obligations, she is being sued by the housing corporation: and she has terminal cancer.

Who thought such a catastrophe could happen two months before retirement.

October 14, 2011

Happy Birthday Mom – it's official – she's a young 80 today!
Sorry folks but this is a long one ...

Help me live: Chapter 8 – "I need to feel hope, but telling me to think positively can make me feel worse."

- Be careful not to extinguish a flame of hope with ignorant and insensitive comments.
- When faced with the realistic impact of mortality there are two ways one could go – you could either say, "You're right and I only have this amount of time" and give up control or latch onto something to give a glimmer, a spark of hope.
- People hope naturally.
- True hope has proved as important as any medication prescribed.
- Just because I cried a lot did not mean that I gave up hope.

- The freedom to experience all our feelings without being judged, without having to hide our doubts, makes hope possible.
- I know I'm going to die and I don't want to waste time thinking about it.
- Talking about the future in a natural way is helpful because it's assuming I will be around.
- Optimism is very different from hope. An optimist says everything's going to turn out just fine. Hope is a feeling; a deeper emotion.
- What's the danger of encouraging someone to look on the bright side? If you believe that your recovery depends on your attitude, then you feel this terrible pressure that negative thoughts could cause your cancer to come back. Also "How can I be positive when I'm so miserable?" It takes energy.
- It's so easy to tell someone to think positive and walk away.
- The failure to think positively can weigh on a patient like a second disease. You think there is something wrong with you if you start feeling bad.
- Feeling despair is normal.
- Insisting that people think positively may even endanger their health. "We want people to say when they are depressed and don't feel good – or else we are not going to be able to help them." They can lose opportunities for genuine intimacy with their loved ones.
- ... and if you think positively then you have a better chance of getting well. It's blaming the victim. Not only do they have to suffer the pain of the cancer, the fear that they're going to die, and the pain of treatment, but also the reality that they will be seen by others in a negative light if they don't get better.
- "You just have to think positively!" is frustrating to hear. You find yourself feeling depressed with intermittent crying jags and people want to blow rainbows up your rear (good one!).
- It's difficult to hear from others that you need to stop feeling sorry for yourself at times when you are depressed or need to cry.

- Being positive, in the midst of incredible odds against you, is just a willingness to get out of bed, brush your teeth, comb your hair (if you did not lose it all) and face the day that awaits you.
- Hope killers – the view of illness as a punishment. This is not happening because you did something wrong, thought negatively or led a stressful life.

Although suggesting that one think positively can have the opposite effect, you can keep it positive by refraining from sharing bad news about the world, news that could instill fear and anxiety, cast out hope and trigger an adrenaline-powered fight or flight reaction.

Easy to remember tip – to foster hope, encourage humour when appropriate, and no cancer horror stories, ever. See you soon.
Nicole XO

Some of us gather at Denise's in the Laurentians to celebrate Mom's 80th birthday. Carmen's energy is limited but she makes the effort to attend. She wears a bulky sweater to hide her weight loss. Every breath is an effort. Her chest rises and falls as she breathes from her upper lungs. Her breathing is shallow. It hurts to see her struggle for air. Family is together and that's important for her and for us all.

October 16, 2011
Good morning. Me again. Just catching up …

Help me live: Chapter 9 – "I want you to respect my judgment and treatment decisions."

- Not helpful – "Maybe you should stop drinking diet pop and try these special vitamins that worked for my cousin …"
- To be trusted is a greater compliment than being loved.[6]
- Some believe your thoughts shape your reality; there are some realities so strong that they persist no matter what.

---

[6] George MacDonald

- I am doing the best I can under the circumstances and will not accept any discussions about things that cannot be undone or changed, and that are not helping me in any way.
- Complimentary therapies, homeopathic therapies, acupuncture, mushrooms, healing science practitioners, etc. Reconciling what you think you know with what the person with cancer wants.
- I don't want people to think of me as sick because that will keep me sick. How people think of you affects who you are.
- When a loved one has cancer … you can't make the decisions or take charge of the problems (even me sis!) … premise all your words and actions on your belief that … you respect their right to choose how they handle their crisis. Make it clear … they are in control of how much you help, and that you will respect their wishes.
- When we hear that someone we love has cancer, we fear for them and also ourselves. We may fear losing our beloved or the life we share with them. Keep in mind that it's about our loved one now and not about us.

It is their life and they have a right to live it their way.

Recognizing and respecting your limits in their lives is one of the ultimate expressions of love (wow – what wisdom!). Nicole XO

★ ★ ★

People are well intentioned.

"Remember the potion I ordered from New Brunswick? The dried herbs product you mixed with water?" Carmen asks.

"Yes. The one you ordered for Dad. It had a bitter taste but he drank it anyway, for a while," I respond.

"It was all a gimmick. You try products thinking they may cure your cancer but they don't."

Carmen had heard the product could save lives. It's not uncommon to receive comments from individuals, some informed and others not, on alternative medicine.

A distant cousin informs us that research is underway at Ottawa University on vaccines against cancer. Carmen discovers herself that she is not eligible for the clinical trials because of her type of cancer.

A volunteer at the hospital claims acupuncture has cured many cancers. The Chinese immigrant comes highly recommended. People line up for hours outside his office, waiting for an appointment. It's first come, first serve. Carmen is in line with George at 7:30 A.M. After an hour wait, Mr. Chang examines my sister and reveals his assessment.

"There is nothing I can do for you. Do not waste your money."

Months later, Carmen refuses the help of a naturopath from Sudbury. He wants to sell her a product to be taken daily without examining her, without knowledge of her medication and medical condition.

October 16, 2011 from Denise
… Carmen called and said she enjoyed her visit and thought it was great the way we organized the food for Mom's birthday party. She is a bit anxious for the week ahead. See you soon xxxx

October 17, 2011
Well, I think we had a fantastic weekend. Short and sweet. I was not too tired yesterday but I did not sleep last night, don't know if it's worries or was just overtired. I will have to check into that later. Love you all so much. Have a nice day. Carmen

October 18, 2011
Well, I did not sleep too well. I think Thursday is making me very nervous. I feel I will need a pail. Of all things, the casino sent me coupons to put in a box twice a week and George went and dropped them off, and I won the VIP night. Of course it's after chemo but I don't care – I will go in a wheelchair if I have to. Carmen

October 19, 2011
Well, good morning. It's not a good one for me. I have not slept well. Today I feel anger not at the world but at how powerless I am with all this shit. Sometimes I wish I could get a really good cry. It happened only once, maybe it's better that way. Well, today

I will be cleansing my soul. I have invited God and everybody up there in my house to pray and to let them know I'm not a happy camper. I guess He is used to that but it will be my first time for a meeting of that kind. I am very nervous for tomorrow. Would like to hide in a hole. Hope I hear what the doctor has to say or will I just pretend that nothing exists, you know we can play that game.

Nicole, I do cry when I think of everything you do for me. I sure hope you don't think I'm ungrateful. I would not even be where we are now if it were not for you, and I will never be able to repay you. I know you don't expect anything in return but I feel so powerless. Please don't quit. Thank you so much for being my friend, sister, bosom. I love you all and am grateful for everything everybody is doing for me. By the way, are the chapters done? I am on withdrawal. Love you all.

My reply
Pay me back? You just have ... you would do the same for me. That's what bosom sisters are for. I know we all feel like we can't do enough ... because we love you.

Have a good meeting. Let it all out, give it all you've got ... but leave a door open!

See you later sis.

Joanne
OK ... you all know what I look like when I cry! After reading these two emails ... I now have to stay in my office for a while until I look normal again. I too wish I could do more ... I love love love you!!!

Sam (a brother-in-law)
OK. I am also with you and feeling it. Let's stick together and keep in touch. Sam. Love you

Carmen
Some may do more than others and I know you work, some are far but I do know I have all your love and support and that means a lot. Love you

October 19, 2011
Hello everyone,
I skipped a few chapters because I found this one more timely and appropriate given what Carmen is going through today.

Help me live: Chapter 24 – Cancer through the stages.

The needs of people with cancer change over time and through treatments.

Soon after diagnosis and before treatment:

- We experience shock, fury, and terror that most of us have never felt before.
- We may feel trapped and immobilized because so much remains unknown.
- Fear paralyzes. That's its nature. When an antelope senses a lion's presence, its nervous system sends out a signal, and it freezes ... when our lives are seriously endangered, we experience a strange paralysis of body and mind.
- Our minds are too muddled to function in an even remotely normal fashion.
- A true trauma, cancer changes us in ways almost impossible to describe. Something has happened to us that goes against everything we ever believed would ever happen to us.
- We feel guilty, angry at our body's betrayal of us. Deeply lonely, our feelings may be volatile, changing quickly and frequently.
- We fear not only death, but disability and the loss of independence. We fear the unknown.
- Because we know so little, asking persistent and repeating questions can be terrifying. Never a good idea to ask too many questions of cancer patients – let them take the lead.

What a newly diagnosed patient needs is love, patience, support, a shoulder, a hand, reassurance, a listening ear and a kind eye. A patient also needs a quiet time alone to listen to their heart and head and have one good sob session (I think this is how Carmen feels today).

Chemotherapy:

- Many with cancer fear chemotherapy more than other treatments and sometimes more than the cancer itself.
- Everyone is different and reacts differently to medications and treatments. Some have side effects and others don't. It varies with each individual.
- Chemo may preclude further suffering and save lives but it can affect the intestinal tract and stomach by killing normal fast-growing cells, causing nausea, vomiting and hair loss. Maybe rashes.
- Sometimes chemo can feel like the worst imaginable flu.
- During chemo it hurts to hear, "It's only hair." Don't pull my wig. Don't tell me chemo is poison and toxic. Respect my choices.
- Don't tell me I look good when I really feel and look bad.

October 19, 2011
You know, a bit more and I will start thinking you can read my mind. So happy you are doing this. I guess that is how I really feel today. I have cried a few times and still am. Anyway will have to stop this shit and get back on the positive side. Just like in *Gone with the Wind* ... too tired, I will think about it tomorrow.
Love Carmen

I read the book, *Help me live*, in its entirety and prepare my summaries. Timing is everything. I choose which chapters to send based on Carmen's emotions and which one I think will be helpful to her. On occasion, I take the liberty to integrate my own comments into the summaries where appropriate. It is not deceitful. The intent is to help her understand her journey. She does not have any interest in reading books regardless of the topic. She does not want to participate in a support group. Her concentration level is low. It is the closest I can come to sharing her experience.

October 19, 2011
Hello Aunt Carmen,
I want to share with you this poem, which was helpful to me in the past. We all know that chemo is difficult and if you take the decision to try it, then read this poem daily for motivation. We are all with you. We love you very much Adam xxx

Never abandon (Anonymous)
When your road is full of obstacles
And that you expect no miracles
You are permitted to rest
But never abandon
When success is out of reach
And self-doubt invades you
Maybe without your knowledge
You are closer to your goal
Only when you have tried everything
… You must never abandon

October 20, 2011 from Carmen
What a day. Slept 30 minutes on the hour. I guess, not too bad. Remember the movie *Shrek* where the cat makes his big sad eyes, wish I could do that so the doctor might not be so hard on me. I will ask Nicole once we are done to send all of you an email with the updates of our meeting. I have put her in charge; she likes to be the boss and for once I really don't mind. My eyes drip every ten minutes, so maybe I will have the puffy eyes when I go. Anyway I love you all and thank you everyone for your support.

The five of us agree to meet in the waiting room of the oncology department. Carmen sits next to her daughter Lisa. George and I sit across facing them. Lisa's face is tense. The fear of the unknown is evident. We all carry the same look. We anxiously make small talk while we wait for Martin's arrival. Carmen is pleased to see her son walk in. I ask him if he cried last night – we all laugh – Martin's eyes are still red and his eyelids are swollen. He hardly slept.

The waiting room is full. We keep busy observing other patients and their families as we wait. I walk from table to table perusing the pamphlets on services available for cancer patients. I don't find much.

My heart skips a beat when I hear the nurse call Carmen's name. Her oncologist is ready to see her. I let them attend as a family and I wait anxiously for their return. When they do, they all seem more relaxed. Carmen likes his bedside manner. She is relieved.

October 20, 2011
Hi everyone,
Based on the results of Carmen's biopsy, the oncologist is not certain if the lungs are the primary or secondary site for the cancer. They have a suspicion the cancer may have started in the ovaries or stomach. They have to do more tests to determine the initial source – which has an impact on the type of chemo she will receive. She is scheduled to meet with her oncologist on November 22nd for the new results and should start her treatments on November 24th.

The biopsy also indicated she has the non-small cell cancer – it grows more slowly than the small cell one.

In the meantime, she's getting ready for her VIP gala at the Casino Lac-Leamy which is in a few days. She may just win the top prize of 10K! Hugs to all. Nicole XO

October 22, 2011
Managed to sleep a good five hours in bed. Well, today I am a bit sad because I think everybody is putting their life on hold for me. Nicole and Roger who always take trips, haven't planned anything. Mom and Tim don't know if they should leave. Nobody is talking about taking holidays. You have to keep the same lifestyle you used to do, okay, maybe a few changes. George has been very good for me; there is nothing he would not do. I think he realizes now I do need space. I feel guilty some times because I don't want

him to think I don't want him, but sometimes I need to be by myself. I'm always scared of hurting people's feelings. Those who live close – maybe we could plan a bowling day even if I throw only one ball. It's just we would be all together. Well, I guess that's all for today. Love you all and thank you all for being there. Love your sister, aunt, mother, friend etc … Carmen :)

My reply
That's good. You need to go out. As for me – it's hunting season. I have to wait until Roger is done with the moose … the deer and … the caribou … or I go on a trip by myself. So it's OK if I'm here waiting for him because I have you to look after :)

Don't forget you and I are due to go west. Nicole

Carmen's reply
Okay sis, you can go on a trip but not too long. Sorry.

October 22, 2011
Hello everyone,
We may need to get organized at this end so people don't burn out. We need to help George. He is the primary support. He does so much.

Help me live: Chapter 19 – "I need you to offer support to my caregiver, because that helps me too."

- Cancer patients are more grateful than they can say …
- When friends called to bring meals over and asked which day would work for us, I cried. Not only was it a show of support but it relieved my wife of something else to deal with.
- Problems begin to set in after two to three months of care giving. You deal with the outer physical aspects of care giving; cooking, cleaning … it can be difficult but you either do the extra work or hire someone to do it.
- What's more difficult is the inner turmoil that starts to accumulate on the emotional and psychological levels. It is twofold; one private and one public. On the private – you stop talking

about your personal problems. You don't want to upset your loved one; make it worse for them. Problems can magnify ... anxiety creeps in ... death hangs in the air; and anger, resentment and bitterness also creep in along with guilt about having such feelings.
- Sooner or later, the caregiver finds out that almost everybody not actually faced with the problem on a daily basis starts to find it boring or annoying that you keep talking about it.
- Caregiving can have an incredible toll on the body and spirit. Caregivers face inevitable stresses and burdens that place them at risk for psychological and physical problems. It ranges from a diminished immune response; cardiovascular, musculoskeletal or abdominal diseases and depression.
- Caregivers need to find coping strategies that work for them. Maybe time to meditate, engage in other activities involving self-care. They need to acknowledge the pain, absorb it and most importantly, let it go (I hope they have a chapter on that one!).
- When one is sick; two need help.
- One of your biggest fears is that your caregiver will burn out. You want them to look after themselves and find support.
- Sometimes our expectations of loved ones are too high. Somehow we feel they should know what to say or do. Know that we are trying to understand how the other feels.
- Sometimes, we need to go back to Chapter One. Nobody is perfect. Forgive.
- Caregiving is on-the-job training.

When an individual has cancer, it's like the whole family has it (I just can't say enough about this book). Talk to you soon. Love Nicole XO

October 23, 2011
Good Morning everyone.

Today I feel great. I have a lot of energy – I feel like a peacock, don't know when the feathers will fall but I will take it while it lasts. But because I'm feeling a lot better Lisa and I started my list again. For those of you who don't know, Lisa always laughed at my list. I write every section in the house and when I am done cleaning one, I scratch if off. Now don't forget, I only started writing things down: it does not mean I will follow it if the feathers drop. I like being a bit of a hoarder I guess. Well, have a nice day everybody. Love you all. Carmen

October 27, 2011
Hello everyone,

Here's the latest update – Carmen saw her family physician earlier this week. Looking at her chest X-rays for the last two years, he concluded her cancer is recent.

As for the walk for lung cancer, it will be held on Saturday November 5th at 8 or 9 A.M. I'll send a separate email to those who are walking to confirm the time and meeting place. We are too late to register as participants but we can contribute to Carmen's colleagues' fundraising campaign. The funds will go to the US to help with cancer research.

Back to the chapters ...

Help me live: Chapter 10 – "I want you to give me an opening to talk about cancer, and then take my lead."

- Sometimes I'm not in the mood for cancer-chat.
- Learn to take the communication lead. If the person is having a good day – let them bring up the subject of health.
- And when they bring up cancer – shut up and listen.
- Sometimes you just want to be normal and play battleship (I want a rematch sis – I still say you cheated!:)).
- Emotions never tell you their cause. You need to talk about it.
- Sometimes it can be impossible to know what a person with cancer wants or needs. Some may resent that you don't ask about their health (how are we to know?).

- Keep it about the person with cancer. Put yourself in their shoes and their heart.

See you soon. Nicole XO

October 31, 2011

Carmen authorizes her office to release all information to me so I may follow up on matters of employment benefits on her behalf. It's getting too complicated for her. She does not have the energy for lengthy discussions. Her appetite is diminishing. She is weak. She sleeps more and is missing important phone calls. Her concentration level is low; it's difficult for her to focus and make decisions. Ordinary things become overwhelming.

When you are emotionally involved it's difficult to make sound decisions on matters you are not familiar with. Dealing with her office is at times demanding. The two individuals I deal with are very pleasant and compassionate; however, on occasion they give me contradictory information. As a result, I doubt their competence and authority. I take copious notes and email a summary of our every discussion. With every summary I ask for a confirmation; never to be received. I consider my communication as a record on file. I hold on to all until they complete my sister's file. It took over nine months to receive a written confirmation from Carmen's employer on the final cost of her benefits. Policy changes and other matters contributed to the delay. Although it was a lengthy process, they were quite generous with my sister.

With their assistance we complete the relevant documentation for the insurance companies. Every insurance company has their own forms and particular process. To my surprise, the insurance company responsible for the long-term disability actually has it in their contract with the employer that employees must also apply for Canada Pension Plan disability or, in my sister case, the Quebec Pension Plan. The amount the employee receives from the government is deducted from the amount to be paid by the insurer. In other words, the insurance company forks out much less for the monthly long-term disability and the patient has yet another bureaucracy to deal with. The challenge is obtaining physicians to complete the insurance and government forms. Some physicians resist, they promise but don't deliver. They are busy and it's time consuming. It's also precious time taken away from direct patient care.

You discover the documentation can only be completed once all test results are in. That can take months. As per my sister's experience, one medical test leads to another before the final results are available.

I leave no chance for additional delays. I hand-deliver, courier or pick up all insurance and government forms to accelerate the process.

I can't imagine how one looks after their own affairs when one is seriously ill. In my sister's case, the outcome is positive. I wonder what happens to those individuals who have cancer and little support. Their precious energy is too depleted to meet the challenges regarding income and benefits.

Some individuals find it unusual that I am looking after my sister's affairs given the age of her children who are in their early thirties. I don't. I never think about whose role it is – I simply do it. Carmen nicknamed me "The Boss" many years ago. It just seems to happen naturally. Besides, Lisa and Martin are working and I am not and I'm more familiar with bureaucracies.

★ ★ ★

The hospital dietitian informs us that cancer cells grow at a much faster rate than normal cells. As a result, Carmen is experiencing fatigue, loss of appetite and dehydration. George and I follow her suggestions; small meals and frequent snacks; for example, "Boost" and "Ensure" drinks provide additional calories; cream soups, juices and Jell-O are helpful for rehydration. Carmen is somewhat resistant. I understand; she has no appetite.

> **November 2, 2011**
> Hello everyone,
>
> Carmen has been very tired lately – she's not sleeping well. She is fatigued, nauseous, has headaches, no appetite; all typical symptoms for people in her condition. Just in case you are thinking of giving advice, the next chapter is on how not to ... now that should be easy-peasy!
>
> Carmen underwent a gastroscopy this afternoon and the good news is she does not have cancer in the stomach. It was clean as

a whistle. Her next medical is a CT Scan next week. As she says, she's never been so busy.

Hope you are enjoying this wonderful weather. Love with a hug, Nicole

Help me live: Chapter 11 – "I want compassion, not pity."

- Humans are the most social of animals. Sometimes we don't want to say we have cancer because we don't want to be cut off from the herd.
- We do not want to be alone and we do not want to feel alone.
- People with cancer need compassion, not pity. We need constructive interactions.
- Sometimes I saw judgment in people's eyes. When people said, "I used to smoke too." I felt a sameness, a sense of compassion, like they knew they could be in the same boat.
- Being ill makes one feel alone.
- Compassion is a relationship between equals ... it becomes real when we recognize our shared humanity.
- The word "pity" can sound condescending.
- I sometimes felt like I had to be strong and keep up a good face because I did not want people to feel sorry for me.
- Allowing someone to feel their pain and feeling their pain with them can seem dangerous but you don't have to let someone else's pain damage you. You can experience it and let it go. Some caregivers cannot release the pain because they want to control it. It's not possible to control. Make it go away. Open yourself up by allowing yourself to imagine what the other person is experiencing. And let it go.
- Compassion leaves no room for judgment and condescension.
- I don't know how you feel. I can only imagine what you are going through.
- "I love you," and "you mean so much to me," meant a lot to hear.

- When you see someone with cancer, look beneath and beyond. And then send love and prayers and good thoughts and hope for healing.
- And as you thank God that it is not you, realize that it could be.

Carmen's reply
Thank God for my sister who does so much for me. I know you would all help if you were close and retired, so don't say I could do more, I understand. I know you are thinking of me and love me as I love you all. I'm feeling very under the weather, trying to go under the radar but it's not working. I can't pretend I don't have it since my body and mind won't let me forget. Poor George tries so hard to please me but imagine how difficult I was before. I guess he will get a straight road to heaven, no bumps. I don't know if I am ready for chemo – sometimes I would just like to lie in a hospital bed and let the nurses take care of me. I would not be a burden on anybody except for Nicole, who can't stop so she can get some green stuff coming in.

I will try to see you on Saturday for those who walk. I have a doctor's appointment at 10:10 A.M. for the flu shot and then I will go where you park your cars and will try to join you for breakfast. Hope I will be feeling okay. If your cars are gone, I will call Nicole or somebody on their cell. Love Carmen.

My reply
Stop that, I don't do much. But ... I do have a list for us to work on today :) Yippee!

November 3, 2011

George wants my sister's health restored. The more he imposes healthy eating, the more Carmen resists. She recognizes the tension in his face and nervousness in his actions. She is aware her emotional moods and impatience make him anxious, nervous and confused. He doesn't know what to do.

Carmen becomes frustrated. Meals are the "BIG" issue. She does not like George's cooking and his recipes. She wants her regular meals. She wants to eat what she wants to eat. The dependency is evident. She becomes angry and nasty.

That afternoon, we plan a weekly menu. The chefs are committed – Lisa, Martin, George and I will take turns preparing her meals. We will prepare what we can at home to prevent her feeling nauseous from cooking odours.

Carmen prefers her autonomy but given her condition our plan is the next best thing. Tired, she spends the rest of the afternoon and evening on her couch sleeping with the television's piercing sound.

That night George dials 911. Carmen has difficulty breathing. Her tumors are growing.

PRAY FOR ME I AM TERRIFIED

November 4, 2011
Hello everyone,

Just so you know, Carmen called the ambulance last night. Her oxygen saturation was at 79% (It is usually around 97% - 99% in a healthy individual). The doctor told her she would remain in the hospital until they can organize and deliver an oxygen tank to her apartment. Given that it's Friday, she may be in the Emergency Department for a few days unless they can do this over the weekend.

She is extremely tired and very weak. They tell her she needs to rest. I don't want to tell you not to phone her – please know it's not my role and I surely do not want to take that responsibility. But to give you an idea, she shared with me that she has 15-20 calls a day. That's a lot of ringy-dingy! All from people she loves. Sometimes she answers, sometimes she doesn't because she is simply too tired to talk.

I will keep you posted as I get news. I have not spoken to George as I know he is tired too. Take care. Love Nicole XO

November 4, 2011 from Lisa
Hey, just got a little bit of news from Martin who talked to George.

Mom is OK, but she is pretty out of it. They gave her some medication because she had a migraine. They will not release her until she has an oxygen tank at home. They will be doing her CT Scan that was scheduled for the 10th this afternoon in the hope that maybe things will go faster for her treatments. She can have visitors but only one at a time and for a period of 20 min only. So George stays with her for 20 min and then walks around the hospital waiting for his other 20 min to see her. There are no words to say how grateful we are for George :). We know he is tired. Martin and I have offered to do anything he wishes in order to help him and Mom. He says he's OK and promises to tell us if he needs anything. There are also no words to thank Aunt Nicole for all the work you have done to help my mom and being there for her.

Will keep you all posted. Thanks
Lisa xoxoxoxoxoxoxoxoxo

November 5, 2011

A few of Carmen's co-workers organized a walk for lung cancer. We participate, we do it for Carmen. I offer my assistance in organizing the 2012 walk. For whatever reason, I never follow through. There are many walks and fundraising activities for cancer research. All are crucial in making progress to find a cure for cancer. Perhaps more attention should also be centred on reducing our risk. People need to stop smoking.

That same weekend the four sisters are together again, sharing special moments. We cuddle up on Carmen's hospital bed. We look alike; have similar expressions. We are close in height and weight except for Carmen. She was always smaller and half a foot shorter.

Carmen is feeling and looking better now that she is on oxygen. In the few hours we are together, hospital staff come and go. Our conversations are candid regardless of the lack of privacy.

Carmen saw several physicians that weekend. One came by during our visit. He confirms with her that she will begin radiation therapy on Monday. Staff will brief her on the process tomorrow. I observe and silently question his approach. He repeatedly emphasizes to my sister that her lungs are finished and damaged from cigarettes. I wonder about the value of making a patient feel like they brought it on to themselves. Do they need to be reminded that their smoking had an impact? Is it necessary? The damage is done. Rather, should the focus not be on her upcoming journey and end-of-life issues? How many times must they reinforce that she is dying?

"The treatments will be administered only to provide you with a quality of life for the time you have remaining. They won't cure your cancer or prolong your life. You understand?" My sister nods. He leaves shortly after.

I remember a paramedic once told me, "People need to hear the 'dead' word." We all heard it – Carmen has one year to live with no hope for recovery. Enough with the reinforcement please.

Not all physicians demonstrate empathy; actually, we encounter few who do. It becomes evident many do not know how to compassionately deal with dying patients and end-of-life issues. They could use my summaries. Better yet, they should read the entire book.

My sister's new quarters is a standard four-bed hospital room, a large room with a partial wall in the centre. Two beds are set on each side of the wall. The open doorway connecting both sides is blocked with a curtain. I assume it was installed for privacy, although limited. During our visit we overhear several conversations.

Behind the curtain a man is dying. His daughters and girlfriend take turns visiting that day. With each visit, one pressures him to change his will and exclude the others. Everyone wants the house. At one point the poor man cries, "What do you want me to do?"

The four sisters look at each other. No need to speak. We can read each others' minds. How sad it is for all of them to spend their last days together in such a way.

Carmen sheds a few more tears as she shares with us how difficult she finds saying goodbye. It is heartbreaking to hear her ask us to care for her children, and not to forget George.

After our hospital visit, we meet George at Carmen's apartment and the four of us do a thorough cleaning of her home. We change her bed, do her laundry, wash her floors and so on.

There seems to be a lingering old tobacco smell in the kitchen. Denise and I are sniffing everything in sight, like two hound dogs on a mission.

We discover it comes from the cooking range exhaust fan. We are confused. Could someone be smoking in the apartment? Could the smell remain years after Carmen stopped smoking? We remove the fan mesh filters and wash them in the dishwasher.

An envelope grabs my attention as I drop another in a basket of papers to file. The handwriting is that of a child. Every stroke is deep and every letter is round and exaggerated. It looks like mine. Within the envelope are two letters folded in their original state. The lined paper turned faint yellow with the years.

I read both letters. These were written in 1971 when I was 11 years old. It was the year the three youngest in the family moved with my parents to Sturgeon Falls, Ontario and the three oldest remained behind in Touraine, Quebec. We are 400 km apart. In my letters, I share with Carmen how much I love her and miss her. It's heartwarming to see she kept my letters for 40 years. I smile. When she leaves I'll take these back. It will be my souvenir of my sister. That's all I want.

George is cautious and uncomfortable; he does not want us to disrupt Carmen's belongings. He knows this is upsetting for my sister.

Carmen is a clean person but the type of individual who prefers to live in an orderly mess. That's on a good day. Since her illness, she has no energy to clean, no motivation. She has difficulty walking, her clothes litter the floor, papers are not filed. Her living room coffee table is barely visible. All her necessities are close at hand. We find resting on the table, her usual, a glass and jug of water, a box of Kleenex, papers, over-the-counter drugs and prescription medications ranging from creams to pain killers, several inhalers, a bowl of candies, empty wrappers, her two remote controls, a cordless phone if not two.

By bringing some order we think we are helping.

November 10, 2011
Hello everyone,

Carmen is still in the hospital. She looks and feels much better since she is on oxygen. Because the tumors have grown and are pushing on her bronchi making it difficult for her to breathe, the physicians have decided to give her approximately six radiation treatments. She was to start today but it was deferred to maybe next week. She will receive these on a daily basis. She is to remain hospitalized until they are done. She's hoping to get a day pass for Saturday depending on how she feels. The side effects of radiation are fatigue, loss of appetite, sore throat.

In addition, she is being given cortisone to reduce the inflammation in her lungs (they say it's working) and this brings on diabetes as a side effect. Hence, the insulin added to the menu. Apparently, radiation and chemo treatments damage bones – she was given a shot/vaccine of calcium because of her osteoporosis. It is more effective than calcium pills and lasts for one year. It too has a side effect, which I think is diarrhea. I can't remember. No worries, she has another medication that gives her constipation – so it all seems to even out in the end. I'm sure I'm missing a few details … she is scheduled for a PET Scan on Monday. I believe this is to detect changes in her cancer and how it's growing.

All said and done, her spirits are good and she is just as beautiful as ever (other than the occasional bad hair day!). She lost a bit more weight (now 96 pounds). Her panties are getting a bit baggy so she sent George to Wal-Mart to get her the granny kind. What this man won't do for her! Her appetite is good. Maybe she will put on a few pounds. She seems to like hospital food. No Wi-Fi. She misses her emails. She sends her love and hugs to all of you. Here's another chapter. Talk soon. Nicole

Help me live: Chapter 12 – "Advice may not be what I need and it may hurt more than help. Try comforting me instead."

- If I want to eat Hostess Twinkies, well, if it will get me through cancer I will eat them.
- Ask permission before giving advice. It's even more crucial when people are striving to maintain their dignity, independence, and sense of control in a world that may suddenly feel unmanageable.

- I know they love me and want to help but sometimes I feel they are undermining my intelligence and treatment program.
- I don't like it when someone starts a sentence with, "You have to ..." I loathe people telling me about alternative medicine or giving me unsolicited medical advice.
- Gestures become the most important form of comfort.
- Intentions are good but you don't want people giving you advice and telling you what you should and shouldn't do without understanding your diagnosis. People would tell me eat lots of fruits and vegetables, eating all that would cause nonstop diarrhea after radiation treatments.
- It hurt to hear, "You know cancer is caused by stress ... you should do something about X ... you should ... you should ..."
- Understand this is my journey.

I lean against the windowsill in Carmen's hospital room. I read out loud my most recent email to the family. I pause to give her and George time to laugh. She loves my summaries. She loves that we care.

★ ★ ★

It's Remembrance Day. Roger and I attend the traditional ceremony held at the National War Memorial, a Cenotaph in downtown Ottawa. As we walk from Elgin Street to the "Tomb of the Unknown Soldier" we meet several of Carmen's colleagues. I don't recognize them. I don't know who they are. Roger smiles as he speaks. The others look on.

"Remember the walk?" he says.

"What walk?" I ask.

"The walk for lung cancer." I become the deer in the headlights. Roger goes on, "The one we did six days ago!"

I was never so embarrassed. I walked with these two individuals for a few hours to raise awareness for lung cancer and I did not recognize them. I had no clue who they were. It took me minutes to recall the walk. I'm concerned about myself. I honestly feel as if I am in another world observing someone else's life.

During my next visit to the hospital, a nurse informs us the oncology department is ready to administer Carmen's radiation tattoos. I accompany them to the unit and stay with my sister while she waits. We often talk of nothing. It feels good to be together.

The radiation therapist brings my sister for her prep work. Marks will be drawn on her chest with a marker to indicate the exact spots where radiation will be aimed. In the meantime, I run from one department to another trying to find a physician to complete insurance and government forms. It becomes a tennis match and I'm the ball.

Eventually I'm told, "No. It's not oncology. You need to see the physician on call for your sister's ward."

I return to the nursing station and explain my dilemma. "I'll leave the forms in the doctor's basket. I'll put them on top so it will be the first thing she sees." I thank him and return to my sister's room. Carmen lifts her hospital gown to show me her tattoos. "I will be able to wash these off once my final treatment is completed," she explains. I stay with Carmen for most of the evening.

A new shift and a different nurse is assigned to my sister. We ask about the forms. She mistakenly says, "It's not the physician's priority." Carmen notices my facial expression. She tries to calm me but it's too late, the firecracker is lit.

"It's OK! It's OK!" Carmen says. She is always pleasant with all healthcare workers. She is so good with the staff.

"No, it's not OK." I raise my voice. I'm upset. "You can't go on this way. I look after your affairs. You don't know where you stand financially. You need revenue." I then address the nurse directly; explaining to her the urgency; the impact and the additional stress this is creating for my sister and her caregivers; how it affects her welfare; how it affects her healthcare. She has no revenue. Being sick is costly. I can't be more direct.

Later that night, the physician does her rounds and actually sits and completes the insurance and government forms with my sister. On occasion, Carmen would translate questions into French. It took them well over an hour. It's no wonder physicians charge patients for their time to complete these. She is one of the few physicians caring for my sister who exemplifies compassion.

The next morning when I walk into the hospital room, George and Carmen are smiling. She holds in her hands the completed insurance and government forms. She hands them to me; I briefly look through the documentation. All seems complete. I note the prognosis. I say nothing. I assume my sister has read the forms.

We stay with Carmen while she eats her lunch. George and I then head down to the cafeteria for a quick bite before they close. I leave the forms with my sister. In the elevator I ask George if he's reviewed them. He hasn't. I inform him of the prognosis. He shakes his head.

When we return to the room, I stay with Carmen and George for a while. The forms remain at the foot of her bed. As I'm preparing to leave, Carmen picks them up and browses through them. Her jaw drops. She looks up at me surprised. Her facial expression continues to change. She's disappointed and upset. She tosses the papers back on the bed in disgust. "She wrote one year!" she exclaims, "I have ONE year!"

I'm as surprised as she, but for different reasons. We all knew this, I thought. The physicians kept reinforcing it the last month.

I'm not sure what to say. I pick up the forms and pretend to read them. I then look at my sister "Initially, the physicians told you it would be one to maybe a year and half." I delay my departure until she is better.

According to Dr. Elizabeth Kübler-Ross the five stages of death are Shock, Denial, Anger, Bargaining and Acceptance[7]. Not necessarily experienced in that order. One works through the different stages but does everyone accept it? Although in the last month Carmen has gone from shock to acceptance to anger and bargaining and now back to denial, she did seem to accept it. So did my father when he went through his journey. Maybe they accepted the diagnosis and not the prognosis. Regardless, hope is vital. How else are we to survive?

Later that week Carmen obtains a day pass for the Saturday. She visits her friend Julie who lives close to the hospital. Carmen is the sister she never had. Julie, a cancer survivor, is very appreciative of the support Carmen gave her several years back when she was diagnosed with osteosarcoma, the type of cancer Terry Fox had.

"Let yourself be loved." She says to my sister, "Let others care for you. You always looked after everyone else. Let it be your turn."

---

[7] Kübler-Ross, Elizabeth. *On Death and Dying*. New York: Scribner, 2003. Print

Julie emails a picture of the two friends hugging. Carmen's face is so swollen due to the medication, she doesn't look like herself. I ache every time I see it.

★ ★ ★

Carmen's hands tremble slightly. Probably from physical weakness or the cocktail of medication she's taking. She is aware her handwriting has changed as a result, "Look at my signature. I can't write anymore." And she hands me the form. The involuntary shaking becomes permanent.

Her financial affairs look more promising. The forms are in with the respective government departments and insurance companies, she is now receiving unemployment insurance and we discover Carmen has insurance on her car loan. She was sure she had declined it when she purchased her car. This means she is no longer responsible for the monthly payments and in a year, the car is paid in full. Now that's good news.

I am always amazed with the bureaucratic process and how unresponsive staff can be to their clientele. I visit the local Service Canada Centre on behalf of my sister. I provide them with a copy of her new medical certificate for their files, given the current one expires at the end of the month. Apparently they need her authorization for this. I explain my sister's condition, she has terminal cancer and she is currently in the hospital for radiation therapy. In the hospital you do not have access to the Internet; therefore, she cannot complete her weekly unemployment forms/stamps; she cannot dial Service Canada's toll free number as the hospital telephone system will cut you off as soon as you enter the number one; and a cell phone is prohibited in her room located in an older wing. In addition, she is ill and therefore cannot spend 30 minutes to an hour waiting on the hospital payphone for a representative to discuss these matters. As for their standard authorization form to assign someone else on her behalf, it reads "incompetence". My sister does not want to sign it. She's not incompetent; she simply does not have access to their system.

I ask for a local number and a representative my sister could contact to address her issues. They refuse. It is not possible to give either. I ask for a business card; that's not possible either. The supervisor's first name only is identified on his name badge. His last name is omitted. Given the poor service provided, I understand why they initiated a policy of only releasing employees' first names. Most insurance companies do the same.

I can appreciate the frustrations people experience dealing with insensitive employees and their uncollaborative, unresponsive processes. It could easily turn out to be life threatening for staff, particularly when a person's mental state is delicate and their livelihood is at stake. Are they contributing to the problem? You wonder how these employees obtain any level of job satisfaction. Surely their values and the company's must conflict, or maybe they don't. Again, I question how people who have no support deal with these situations. How many give up? What hardship follows as a result? My heart cries out for them.

November 16, 2011
Hello everyone,

Here's the latest. Carmen is undergoing her radiation treatments daily. She is experiencing a few side effects, which may increase with every treatment. She may feel it more tomorrow or Friday. She is not as energetic as this past weekend. She is tired, now has mushrooms in her mouth (not the kind you buy at Loblaws!) probably from the drugs.

She had a few accidents yesterday as she was walking around in the hospital – another side effect. And so Carmen is now wearing Pampers. They first tried Depends but they were too big. When you think it's gas, it may not be. She's thrown out three panties so far. I guess George will be heading to Wal-Mart again! Her butt is on fire and she already has gone through one pot of cream. She wants me to share everything!

Carmen is a bit more fragile. She is living through the biggest stress in life, yet sometimes it's the smaller things that make her cry or overwhelm her. We give her great big hugs and lots of love. It's not fair – she does not deserve this – no one does.

She may be going home on Friday or Saturday. We will keep you posted. She sends her love and so do I. Take care. Nicole

P.S. I've added Carmen's dearest friend Louise to our mailing list.

Help me live: Chapter 13 – "I am still me; treat me kindly, not differently."

- Cancer changes most people profoundly in ways that defy description. Even though you can't see nor be the old you, you don't want to be treated differently.
- When we see a sick person as a patient, we undervalue their strengths. When sick, you are unusually vulnerable to the opinions of others so if we see someone as a helpless victim, they are likely to see themselves the same way.
- Cancer does not make me a hero. Cancer does not make you strong.
- My husband did not fuss over me when I attempted to do things I probably shouldn't have done, he just allowed me to do things as normally as possible.
- People don't change when they get cancer and don't stop wanting to be called smart, sexy, funny, an excellent cook, singer, etc. People are more than their cancer.
- You still need to do certain things for yourself. I want to cook when I can.
- Treat us like we are still normal. Don't look at us with pity in your eyes or voice. Don't be patronizing.
- People with cancer are people first.

Looking back, those were difficult times. My sister trusted me with her affairs but I could sense her stress. It seems every time I see her I have forms or letters for her signature. One time I sit next to her on her hospital bed so we may review another government form together. She questions my approach and the content; I try to explain the process but it's complicated. I'm tired of arguing and abruptly say, "Then tell me what you want me to do!" She begins to cry. It quickly turns to sobbing. I'm holding her tight in my arms. She is so skinny and fragile; I feel her shoulders jerk with every sob, her body shaking with tears. I don't remember seeing her cry this much, ever. I'm sorry I'm so impatient and insensitive. She's sorry she can't handle it all. George is sitting in the chair silently watching. My sister is powerless, another loss of autonomy. No words can adequately describe how I feel that day.

Future outbursts will occur but with different individuals.

★ ★ ★

A sign on the windowsill outside my sister's apartment reads, "Danger. Oxygen in use. No smoking or open flame".

Next to the front door sit eight oxygen cylinders and a cart tank holder with two small wheels. These will be used for Carmen's outings. They are to be replenished every Tuesday to guarantee a supply of oxygen in case of a power failure.

The oxygen concentrator (a large apparatus on wheels that has to be plugged in to generate oxygen) is also a permanent fixture. It stands in the hallway, halfway between my sister's bedroom and her living room. The plastic nasal tubing is long enough for her to walk to any room in her apartment. The constant rhythmic purging sound it generates competes with the television.

George phones me. Carmen was discharged from the hospital. They are at home. I hear my sister in the background. I can't make out what she is saying but by her tone of voice I know she's upset.

"Did you move any papers when you last cleaned the apartment?" he says nervously.

"I don't think so."

"She can't find the bank documents with her password. They were in the third drawer of her dresser in her room."

"Yes. Now I remember. It was the only thing in the drawer. I'm not sure exactly where I put them. I moved them to put clothes away. I did not realize the document included her password. Check the basket in her storage room on top of the dresser. Maybe that's where I put them, with her other papers."

Carmen hates it when we touch her belongings. I don't need to be there. I can picture it. I know she is taking it out on George. Again, it's not his fault.

As stated by Barbara Okun and Joseph Nowinski, there are five stages of family grief namely Crisis, Unity, Upheaval, Resolution and Renewal[8]. We are currently experiencing the upheaval stage. We will be here for a while. We try, we feel helpless and incompetent with this disease and its power over all of us. We are scared and we hurt. I believe all are expressions of our innocence.

November 20, 2011
Hi everybody,

I am back home, a bit tired but the radiation went well. They said my body took it very well. I feel a bit stronger every day. Had a nice evening last night with Nicole and Joanne. Believe it or not, Nicole is really getting to be a cook. Excellent meal. Next week I will meet the oncologist for the chemo. I will have to see about the side effects before I confirm, as they said it will not extend my time. I love you all and can't thank you enough for everything you guys are doing. Like I said to Nicole and Joanne, I want to control my cleaning which I was no expert at to start off with, but I want to do my own things while I can. I will maybe need somebody once I start chemo. I do not wish to put everything on George, he's busy shopping for Pampers or panties and he has a cold. The phone rings less and of course, I love receiving calls from my family. If I don't answer, it is because the phone is not near me or I am sleeping but will call back don't worry. Love you all. Carmen

November 21, 2011
Well, it's 3:30 – I think I have a ghost with a heater in my bed and he puts it under my covers so I can perspire a lot. I wake up all wet and of course, I lift my arm to move, well the smell that comes out of the armpits is enough to kill a safari. Of course, I can't use perfume so here I am washing body parts especially armpits. Did you know I have not had a real good shower or bath,

---

[8] Okun, Barbara and Joseph Nowinski. *Saying Goodbye: A Guide to Coping with a Loved One's Terminal Illness.* New York: Berkley books, 2011. Print.

like I mean scrub a dub, since September? Just parts of my body because of my PICC line. God, the things we take for granted. Well, I guess I will try to go back to sleep now. Good night everybody. Love you. Carmen

My reply
A close family shares everything!

★ ★ ★

Roger agrees to accompany Carmen to the casino. It's a trip away from Cancerland. George and I are not invited – we are regarded as the two black clouds.

"She is so frail. You blow on her and she may keel over." Roger is paranoid about Carmen's displacement. I give him a few tips on how best to proceed.

The morning news is on. Carmen is sitting on her couch holding her purse, impatiently waiting for Roger's call. The phone rings. She listens for the code, "I'm just about to cross the bridge."

"I'm ready." She quickly hangs up and turns off the television.

She manoeuvres her oxygen nasal tube to avoid tripping as she quickly makes her way to the washroom one last time.

Roger parks the car at her front entrance and turns on the passenger seat warmer. As he walks to the front door my sister looks through the window. She's excited. She opens the door and points to an oxygen cylinder. Under her supervision, Roger inserts it in the designated cart, attaches the plastic nasal tube, slowly opens the cylinder valve and sets the flow gauge to 1.5. He carries the cylinder to the car and places it in a standing position behind the passenger seat. He positions the nasal tube between the two front seats, making it easily accessible to my sister when she gets in.

Carmen is too impatient to wait for him. She slips on her coat, removes her nasal tube and leaves it resting on the chair with the oxygen concentrator still on. She walks out of her apartment. The door locks automatically behind her.

Roger quickly runs back to help her walk up the three stairs and guides her to the car. The passenger door is open. She slides in and immediately reaches for the nasal tube, clips on her seatbelt. She is good to go.

It's all about logistics. Carmen wants to arrive at the casino before the morning rush. They use the McDonalds drive-through for an Egg McMuffin and a coffee. They eat quickly in the parking lot sitting in the car. They discuss their plan. They agree to a spending limit.

As they arrive at the Casino Lac-Leamy, the attendant greets Carmen with a wheelchair. She presents her VIP card for the valet parking. Roger places the oxygen tank between her legs and off they go.

Carmen's face lights up. She is so excited. She knows which slot machines she wants to play. Roger zips through the alleyways to get there. He has to be fast, she is impatient. Did they get there early enough? They look ahead to see if her favourite slot machine is available. It is!

Carmen sits on the stool to play. The oxygen cylinder is next to her. The wheelchair is close by. She ignores the occasional stare. She inserts her Casino Privilege card into the slot machine's card reader. She uses the touch screen to enter her Personal Identification Number and the dollar amount to be transferred into credits. She confirms her transaction. She hits the "MAX BET" button and watches the reels spin while looking for a pattern of symbols. When the timing is right, with a quick motion, she touches the screen, alternating with both hands to make it stop. Her touch is quick and aggressive. The machine pays off. Her fingers reach the "MAX BET" button again and she repeats the exercise. She is in a trance.

Roger verifies the gauge to see how much oxygen is left in the cylinder. Both were advised to closely monitor this, not to repeat a previous incident where she barely had enough oxygen left to make it home. They have since learned how to calculate the time remaining.

Carmen can no longer stand the pain in her sitting bones. It's time to leave. She needs rest. She returns to her wheelchair.

She must use the ladies washroom before going home. Roger brings her to the entrance. She does not have the strength in her arms to wheel herself in. She does not want any help from strangers. The oxygen tank is still in its designated cart. It has two small wheels. Roger removes the cart and tank resting between Carmen's legs. He helps her get up. Carmen is able to walk into the ladies room rolling and leaning on the cart for balance. She is alone.

It seems to take forever. Roger is nervous given her condition. He interrupts a woman playing a slot machine. She agrees to go in and check on Carmen, and he offers to wait next to her slot machine to reserve it. Both come out a minute later. Roger is relieved. Carmen did not need assistance.

They proceed with their ritual once Roger returns from the cashier counter. He sets aside a tip for the valet. Carmen sits with the palm of her hands open. They split the winnings – one hand for her, one hand for him. Most times they win. Today they made $1200 each. She plans on giving her children a special gift. He will hold on to his share; it will eventually become part of her future winnings.

On the way home she twists and moves in her seat trying to find a comfortable position. She is in pain. She takes her morphine. As they enter her apartment a neighbour inquires if they won. She nods, grabs the nasal tube she previously left on the chair and removes her coat. She leaves Roger to set aside the portable tank without her supervision. She quickly makes her way to the couch and crashes. She is satisfied.

★ ★ ★

A few days later, George and I escort my sister to another early morning medical appointment. We wait in the general waiting room. My sister is asked to sit in the adjacent room with cancer patients only. All are waiting for a medical consultation. This is my sister's first meeting. She is the "newbie," a face they have never seen. The patients have much in common and much to share.

"What type of cancer do you have?" her neighbour asks.

"What stage are you at?" asks another.

Among them they share cancer stories, their treatments and side effects, what to expect, the "do's and don'ts," advice, and which physicians are kind and caring. They can openly and truthfully discuss all subject matters since family members are not present. They share intimate details.

"I dread these consultations. Every time I have a medical test it reveals my cancer has spread elsewhere. Now it's in my brain. The last time they announced it was in my bones." Claire is in her mid 40s and has a ten-year-old daughter from a previous relationship. She and her common law spouse will get married next week. He will adopt and care for her daughter once she is gone.

"You'll see the same faces for a while and then you don't," Claire returns to her magazine.

Carmen never saw her again.

★ ★ ★

My sister smiles as I hand her a finger pulse oximetre.

"It measures your pulse and oxygen saturation. It's similar to the one our guide used when we climbed Mount Kilimanjaro. It may not look as sophisticated as the one in the hospital but it's just as effective. Try it," I say. Her oxygen is at 98 and her pulse not far behind.

She hands it over to George. The three of us take turns trying out the new gadget.

"OK. We'll wear out the batteries," she says as she makes room for it on the coffee table which becomes its permanent place.

November 23, 2011
Sorry folks – I'm behind schedule!

Help me live: Chapter 15 – "I love being held in your thoughts or prayers."

- Many said they kept me in their prayers – that felt wonderful.
- A friend told me I was wrapped in her love and prayers – I never forgot those words.
- They pray for me every day. I really believe that has helped me survive.
- You need all the ammunition you can gather, not just to fight the cancer but to keep your head and heart above water.
- The more votes the better!
- We are hoping and praying with you that things turn out well, so that you don't have to feel that you are facing this frightening situation alone.
- Prayer can redeem people from isolation.

- For people who don't pray much, it can be frightening when they hear others are praying for them. They associate prayers with death.

It's wise to consider your loved one's belief. No matter what, everyone needs and wants to know that they matter. I love you is the statement most people yearn to hear. And so, I love you too! Nicole

Carmen's reply
How nice. I love you all. Carmen

November 24, 2011
Good Morning everyone,

I know it's four but I slept six hours so I guess that was enough for tonight. I think I have a water fountain in this body that sprays water since I can't take a good shower. Anyway, I just wanted to let everybody know how I feel. I have not felt this good physically since August. I am getting stronger every day, mentally and physically. I sprained an ankle yesterday, so of course, Madame has to limp for a few days. I wanted to share with you the road I am travelling presently. Things might not be said in order but my head is all there, even if the government thinks we are stupid because we are sick. Well, to start off, I find the values of life have changed. I want to thank God and everybody who is praying for me because God did hear you. I did not lose interest in reading, watching TV etc., but I find my mind is more focused on what our priorities in life are. You know, when you are not sick, you do not really find the time to tell everybody how much you love them or visit because we are so busy in our little world and we always find excuses, it's far, we're lazy, stuck watching these programs but for me now, I want quality time with each one of you since I love you all so much and know you all love me. So my brain tries to think what we can do. We are very blessed to have such a wonderful family. Oh, by the way, this is not a five minute crying session, only one of joy to let you know I am doing fine. Okay, I have to add this, I don't know if Nicole is done reading the chapters but I am on withdrawal, maybe she could buy another book. I meet the oncologist on Friday for my chemo, but I have decided I will start them only after December 10 because Martin, Lisa and I have rented a cottage, and I do not want to be sick. I want to have a nice weekend for them. I love you all. Carmen

Carmen needs an outing. The four of us are at the entrance way of her apartment. I am holding the door open; my hands are full with Carmen's purse and other belongings. Roger and George are barely outside the doorway looking after the portable oxygen tanks. To our surprise, Carmen sprints by us for the staircase; she lifts her left leg for the first step but it's not strong enough to support her weight and she begins falling backwards. George runs and grabs my sister just before her back and head hit the floor. It all happened quickly. She simply folded at the knees and fell backward. In the process, she tears a tendon in her ankle and foot.

"What were you thinking?" I shout "You have to wait until we are ready."

"I thought if I tried hard enough I would be able to go up the stairs by myself."

They won't operate on my sister due to her lungs. Her leg and foot become obstacles she will have to live with for the rest of her life – additional pain and less mobility.

November 25, 2011 from Lisa
Hi everyone,

Just sending you all an e-mail to tell you about my mom's doctor appointment this morning and a picture of her new haircut :).

She finally met with her oncologist and got the details for her chemo. Well, first off I have to say they made us wait a long time in the waiting room because they couldn't find her file. The nurse was telling her she should have been in the doctor's office already, but they couldn't find her file and were wondering if it was anywhere else in the hospital … Needless to say, Mom was starting to panic a little bit. Also adding to the stress was the fact she had no idea what her treatments were going to be and when she was going to start them.

She knew she only wanted to start them after December 10th, since Martin and I have rented a cottage to spend some quality time, and Mom wanted to feel good and not be sick from the treatments. Everyone was acting like she had to start her treatments right after her meeting with the oncologist, but she was not mentally prepared for this, not today.

They finally found her file and she was able to meet the doctor. Everything went better than we had expected; he said she could not start her chemo today because she had radiation last week and they have to wait at least two weeks between the treatments. That was a big relief for Mom as she was not ready mentally to start. He said she had to do six treatments of chemo, which also was a pleasant surprise; we had no idea what to expect. It could have been 20 for all we knew. So hearing she had six was a big relief. She has a "big one," they say that because they give her two medications in one and it should last about two to three hours (which was also another relief because some people have treatments that last all day). Then eight days after the big one, she gets a "small one" which is a dose of only one medication and should last for about 30 min :). So in total she gets three big ones and three small ones. The treatments average to about two per month, which gives her time to rest and build some strength back. Her first one is scheduled to start December 14th. The oncologist was such a nice person and very comforting. He said she may be able to travel, but only after her treatments are done. They have to take blood work before each treatment to make sure her blood is ok because she may need blood transfusions. They said the treatments may help her cancer from growing or slow it down and give her more time.

After the doctor, we met with her nurse "Pivot" (she is a nurse who takes care of her while she is having her treatments) – she is the link between Mom and the doctor. She's also very nice.

She asked my mom questions about her medical history to know how she was doing mentally and how she was dealing with all of this. She said my mom will lose some hair but not all, it will be thinner, but she will not lose her eyebrows or eyelashes. After an hour in her office, we had finally answered all of her questions. When we were on our way out the door, she told my mom she wanted to congratulate her as she had never met anybody with such a positive attitude and what a great role model she was for her children :). We left there and we are really happy that everything went so well.

Mom, I can't tell you how proud I am of you :), you did your radiation treatments like a champion and you truly are an inspiration to all of us, and I am so proud to say I am your daughter xoxoxoxoxoxxo

Thanks everyone for all of your help, love and support. Lisa

Carmen's reply
Thank you so much Lisa. You and Martin are my pride and joy and the greatest gift I received in life. Love you so much. Carmen

November 29, 2011
Well, good morning everyone.

I have been quiet for a while. Martin came last week and said "Mom, you know I haven't had frog legs in years." So I decided to make him his favorite supper last night. Felt good to smell the food I was cooking instead of reheating all the time. Martin and George changed my bed. We had a great meal. But the farts coming out I thought I was sleeping in a swamp. Everything is fine mentally but I think radiation this week is making me a bit more tired, sleepy. I will relax this week as I am meeting all my co-workers for our Christmas supper Friday and I really want to go; 21 years with them. I can't wait for next weekend with my two adorable children; it will be the best time we will have, it's all about love. Anyway, I love you all and please keep the prayers going because I know God is listening. Thank you.

On my next visit to Carmen's, I'm surprised to find her cooking on the stove. "It smells good. What are you cooking?" I ask.

"Onions – it's to hide the smell."

"What smell?"

"Gas – I'm bloated and I have gas. I can't stand myself."

"Side effects of the medication?"

"Yes. A cancer patient told me to cook onions. It works."

"I'm happy it does." We laugh.

December 1, 2011

Hello everyone,

Carmen has put on a few pounds. She's as cute as a chipmunk! Her cheeks are round (effects of the cortisone) and her feet and ankles are also swollen (effects of radiation) so it looks like she has both ends covered.

Although she has been feeling tired the last few days, her spirits are high. At times she is functioning well without oxygen. She is looking forward to her office Christmas party Friday night. Forget a new pair of shoes or a new dress – she plans on getting a walker for the occasion. She's also excited (and so are we) of her upcoming visit with her close friend Louise who is coming in from B.C. this weekend.

I only have a few chapters left to report on. I may have to think of something else to keep you entertained ... :) Nicole XO

Help me live: Chapter 14 – "If you really want to help me, be specific about your offer or just help without asking."

- I love it when friends called each other about what I needed instead of me having to make the call.
- Instead of asking, "Can I do anything?" Just do something. Don't wait for me or my caregiver to ask, because we more than likely won't.

- She was there if I needed her but she wouldn't be hurt if I didn't.
- Gestures – make them simple and not empty. Follow through.
- Asking someone who is overwhelmed about what they need is not what they need. Food? "Not hungry." Exercise? "I'm running from cancer as fast as I can." Clean clothes? "Oh those …" Be proactive and specific about what you can do.
- On the other hand sometimes we may need to ask permission to help. One of the things people with cancer must cope with is being totally out of control. Arranging their own help may give them control and dignity.

And sometimes they just want to live a normal life and do the simple things themselves. Love, Nicole

December 1, 2011

Well, I guess you will have to get a new book to entertain me. I really loved all these chapters. It was as if I was the one talking. You did a great job. Love you for everything. Carmen

December 2, 2011

Slept well but woke up panicky and excited for Louise is coming down. I want to look my greatest for my supper tonight with my co-workers. I don't really want to look like a chipmunk. I will rest today so I will be in top shape for tonight. I will give you update later. Gotta go feed these cheeks!
Love, Carmen

December 2, 2011

Hi again,

The following is Carmen's chemo schedule for your info. She begins her treatments this month. She's getting six in all; three double doses** and three single doses*.

December 14th**
December 22nd*
December 30th**

January 7th*
January 15th**
January 23rd*
We had great news today. Carmen's long-term disability insurance claim has been accepted. She will be receiving her first cheque December 25th. We don't know for how much yet but at least something is coming in. Nicole XO

December 4, 2011
Well, I have to work on my mind. I am having panic attacks for that chemo. Thank God when we went on trips, the sisters would yap about seven habits or whatever, I guess my brain took some in. I will work on it. Well, back to bed, tired now. Carmen.

Early morning, Carmen sends me this email.

December 6, 2011
Well, the tears are just rolling out of my eyes. I can't stop crying. It's like a faucet, no five minutes, can't stop it. I have to talk to you on a one and one basis which will be confidential. You will be allowed to share it with Roger since he is your other half. Maybe next week or Sunday, when I come back from the cottage with my kids. Thank you so much. I love you lots. I hate it because I can't stop crying. I don't look like a chipmunk now I look like an air balloon waiting for the needle to pop it.

My reply
You decide whenever you want to see me, I'll be there. And if you can't stop crying – then let it all out. You wonder if tear ducts ever go empty.

I love you too, bosom friend. Maybe I can sleep over and we can watch *Murder She Wrote* like the good old days!

By the time we spoke next, Carmen had forgotten what she wanted to share.

December 7, 2011
Well, what a nice surprise from my friend Louise (36 year

friendship which I would never trade for anything). Tears of joy to have seen her. Of course time is short, she will have to go back home but to spend quality time with her is so nice. Louise, we have such a wonderful relationship even if we don't talk often, I know we think of each other. I admire you so much, you don't take life for granted, you savour everything God has given you, nature, friendship, caring for people with respect. Always there to listen but left people to make their decision, you did not try to influence them. Never said a bad word against anybody. I love you so much. You always applied yourself in everything you did and always succeeded. Sometimes I had to push your ass but you made it. I am so proud of you. You do make a difference in this world especially where you are working now. Just tell yourself, if the others don't care as much for the patients, you do compensate for them. We had a lot of chatting to do in a few days. Thank you so much for coming, we are true friends. Love waiting for my next visit.

Carmen expresses her gratitude to family and friends. She knits, with the assistance of a neighbour, scarves for the women in the family. She begins a rag carpet for her friend Julie and crochets a special tablecloth for Denise. Ironically, at the same time Carmen and I give each other a Thank You card expressing our love and gratitude for our special relationship. She sends a touching letter to Mom and she prepares a PowerPoint presentation with photos for her children. Her special thank you letter to George remains a draft. She begins giving souvenirs. She wants to be remembered.

December 7, 2011
Hi sis. Well, it is done because this is what I want to say. Maybe later on I will add to the PowerPoint. I might bring them a copy for this weekend, what do you think? Slept well last night, hard as a rock. Muffin was good, you are getting to be a good cook. I was worried yesterday because my head was confused a few times. I was lost with the PICC line and then, I thought I had slept 24 hours without waking up. Working on my chemo, seemed to work last night. Thinking positive. We will have to go shopping for hats and scarf before I go bald. I know I put a lot of pressure

on you for all the documents, but I appreciate it so much and I like it that you are the boss. The reason I was worried and crying is that I just want to make sure my children are ok and that everything I did was for them. We have to get that leech out of Martin's life so he can start his own business. He has so much potential.

December 9, 2011 to Carmen, Martin and Lisa
Wishing the three of you a wonderful and very special weekend.
May your hearts be filled with love
And your attitudes full of gratitude
May your laughter come from your bellies and resonate throughout the walls and ceiling
And your tears be only of joy
May this time together create special moments to share and cherish forever.
OK, so it does not rhyme and I may not get a job with Hallmark but I'm pretty impressed with myself. Have fun guys! Nicole

From Carmen
Thank you so much. I love you.

Lisa parks her SUV at the front entrance of her mother's apartment. She opens the tailgate and cautiously moves the boxes to make room for the oxygen cylinders and the concentrator. The boxes contain casseroles and food for their special weekend together, just the three of them – mother, son and daughter.

It's a cold day. Lisa runs to Carmen's apartment, her long blond hair flowing in the wind, her breasts bouncing a millisecond after every step. She resembles her mother.

George throws one last sweater into Carmen's duffle bag. He makes his way outside and places it in the back seat of Lisa's SUV. He continues by loading the oxygen tanks. He adds spare nasal tubes for both size oxygen machines.

In the meantime, Lisa helps Carmen into the SUV. George kisses Carmen goodbye and makes his way to Lisa to do the same. It is early Friday afternoon; Carmen and Lisa leave for the rental cottage.

An hour later they reach their destination. Lisa helps her mother out of the SUV and up the stairs into the cottage. They take a quick look around. They will be comfortable for the weekend. Lisa unloads the SUV and brings in all supplies while Carmen supervises. She organizes the cottage for their stay. Martin arrives late that afternoon.

They have a wonderful weekend together, reminiscing about their lives. To their surprise, Carmen delivers her PowerPoint presentation. She tells them stories they heard many times before. They laugh and they cry.

Carmen shares her experience and sorrow when Dad passed away. She tells them, "It hurts but it will get better. After a while, you'll see." She does not speak of fear of dying. She never has. She's just afraid of suffering.

"I'll miss you," Lisa cries.

"I'll be there even if you don't see me."

"Don't freak me out, Mom. If you have something to tell me, tell me in my dreams." They laugh.

Spending the weekend together was an eye opener for Martin and Lisa. They realize the amount of work and effort required to care for their mother. The weekend away is more than lugging clothes and food; it's also the oxygen cylinders, helping their mother up the stairs, preparing her meals, serving her and making her comfortable. They don't sleep well. They are in the country, far from the hospital. They worry when Carmen makes her way to the washroom in the night. They can better appreciate what George does, day in and day out.

December 11, 2011

Hello everyone,

You probably have heard some of these comments; I know I have. And I've actually said some of them myself in the past – Yikes! Now I know better.

Help me live: Chapter 16 – "Hearing platitudes or what's good about cancer can minimize my feelings."

Platitudes are often voiced without thought. They come to mind easily because they have been "tried and true" except when they are not. Such clichés may come across as insincere; they sound generic and don't consider the individual's unique situation.

Some common sayings seem to strike many cancer survivors as inappropriate. The platitudes most disliked are …

- "Any of us could get hit by a car." It's hard to explain that it does feel different from your normal, statistical risk of being hit by a car. This cliché sounds like the person is putting themselves on the same level. We will all die, but the difference is people with cancer may have a better idea of when and are better equipped to prepare and cope for the end. The cliché minimizes the process of what happens along the way.
- "At least …" Even if you get to say goodbye, you don't want others saying, "At least you got to say goodbye." It trivializes a deep and profound loss.
- "You just have to think positively." Reminds you that someone else has it worse and you are in some way lucky!
- "Everything happens for a reason." Sometimes things just happen.
- "Everything's going to be OK," or "You'll be just fine." The statements are meant to encourage but it trivializes the seriousness of the disease. Nobody including the oncologist knows if a patient will be fine.
- "God does not give you more than you can handle." Then what about people who commit suicide?
- "Cancer is a gift." A gift is something you would give away. To whom would you give this gift? What's the return policy?
- "It's God's will." Why would God want me to suffer like this?
- "He's in a better place now." A better place for my husband would be in my arms!
- "I know what you're going through" or "I know how you feel." You don't.

When the words come from someone who cannot truly know what it's like to go through this, the words can be insulting. Be aware that some people have a restrictive range of emotions and cannot deal with bad news or sick people. Let's think twice before speaking …

Nicole XO

December 12, 2011
Well, I really thought the book was done. I had a great weekend with my two adorable children. It was so peaceful – all we did was eat, drink wine and relax. Martin and Lisa did all the cooking, took care of me like a queen. Laughed a lot. Martin says nobody can beat his mom's guilt trip. He tells his friends, "You want to make me feel guilty, go see my mom – she's the queen." We took a few pictures. Martin will send copies.

My reply
I have two more chapters then I'll have to think of something else. Maybe really special quotes. Don't know – need to think about it.

How was the pie? Call me in the morning. Miss you. XO Your bosom friend.

December 14, 2011
Well, I know what the problem is. I sleep all day and am up like an owl at night with my chipmunk cheeks. It's 3 A.M. Let's see if I can sleep more. I will send my agenda for chemo tomorrow. Going into an unknown space, everything will be okay. Maybe we could get people to start praying so I can just zoom through this shit. Good night. Love you all. Carmen

From Ken (a brother-in-law)
The moment I wake up
Before I put on my make-up
I say a little prayer for you.

It's much easier being two to care for Carmen. Apart from her lack of strength, she is extremely impatient. Nothing comes fast enough – except chemo and death. My best description is an aura of impatience, one that instantly amplifies with any medical appointment.

As we arrive at the hospital, George parks the car at the front entrance. They wait for me as I run inside for a wheelchair. Sometimes one is available at the entrance, other times I need to look around.

George helps Carmen out of the car into the wheelchair as I hold and lock it in place. We attach the oxygen cylinder to the back of the chair. We hurry since the cold weather brings a shortness of breath to those with emphysema. We ask Carmen to breathe into her scarf but she doesn't always listen.

While George parks the car in the designated area for cancer patients, I wheel Carmen into the hospital. The wind is cold. We wait at the front entrance for the automated doors to open. They don't. Someone is standing in front of the sensor. We signal them to move; the doors finally open and we make our way to the registration desk. Before standing in line we stop in the ladies room. The quarters are tight with the wheelchair. There's only room for the two of us.

Today will be Carmen's first chemo treatment. She is terrified. They whisk her away for a blood test. George and I stay behind in the waiting room. We choose a small two-seater sofa so Carmen will be able to rest when she returns.

The results arrive an hour later. Her red and white blood cell counts are good. We are given a number and told to bring her upstairs for her treatment. As we enter the room, the nurse informs us that access is limited to cancer patients only. We cannot stay. George waits at the entrance and I follow the nurse's instructions. I wheel Carmen to her chair. The number on the chair coincides with the number given to us earlier.

The room is divided into three sections. Each section has close to eight reclining chairs set up in a semi-circle. The first and second sections are full. Carmen and I gaze at the patients as we make our way through. Most look healthier than expected; some have hair loss; a few have a grey tinge. All are keeping busy doing crosswords, knitting, etc. All have an intravenous. None appear as frail as my sister.

Carmen is the only one in her section, the other chairs are empty. "Other patients will arrive later. If you prefer, I can set you up in the other section so you are not alone." I'm surprised Carmen declines the nurse's offer. It's not like her. She usually likes to speak with other cancer patients and exchange stories.

I help her into her chair and try to make her comfortable. We don't recline the chair; the emphysema, the cancer and stress make it difficult for her to breathe if she leans back. They give her a blanket. On the coffee table I leave her water, a pen and a few puzzles. How I wish I could stay. It breaks my heart that she is going through this. It tears me apart.

The nurse returns and connects the intravenous to her PICC line. She explains the process. They begin with a solution of IV saline fluid. The next IV bag is the chemo. A double dose is prescribed followed by antinausea medicine. The last bag of solution is to flush out her veins before discontinuing the IV. It will take well over three hours. My sister and I kiss and hug. I leave the wheelchair behind. I meet George at the entrance and we return to the waiting room.

It's been over two hours; George obtains a parking voucher for when we leave while I check in on Carmen. I walk directly to my sister's section unnoticed. My poor sister is alone. She is hyperventilating, struggling for every breath. Both her hands are clinging to the arms of the chair as she tries to hold her body forward to ease her breathing. Pulling and holding her body in this position demands a lot of effort and energy on her part. Carmen is hyperventilating so much she can hardly speak to me.

Someone had reclined the chair. I bring it back to a proper position and remove the blanket. She still can't catch her breath. Her eyes are bulging; her jaw and facial muscles are tense. She looks terrified. "Have they not checked in on you? Have they not tried to help you breathe?" She shakes her head NO. She's been in this position for hours.

"You need to relax and slow down your breath." I realize she can't do it. She's drowning.

I kneel next to her. "Let's try yoga breathing. Inhale and exhale from the nose … oh, maybe not sis, I didn't think of your nasal tube. OK. Follow my lead. Inhale from the nose keeping your mouth closed and exhale from the mouth. Make an 'O' with your mouth as you exhale."

We keep eye contact. I exaggerate my breathing motions and sound with every breath … exhale slowly … exhale slowly. Eventually she is able to close her mouth while inhaling. "Just focus on your breath … deep inhale … slow exhale. That's it." It takes a few minutes before she can relax and breathe normally again, her normal shallow breath. I stay with her until the end of her treatment. Her visualization did not work as it did during her radiation therapy; all she could think of was poison entering her body with every drip. She recalls another patient's words, "I've never been so sick in my life. Chemo is worse than the cancer."

I speak to the nurse. It falls on deaf ears. She removes the empty intravenous bag and cleans my sister's PICC line. We wait for the pharmacist to explain the medication and side effects. All is well documented including an emergency number for the pharmacist on call.

Once he leaves, my sister takes her medication. She does not follow his instructions and wait until she is nauseous. She follows the advice given to her by other cancer patients, "Take it now. Once you vomit, it's too late."

I help her into her wheelchair. She is totally worn out. Another traumatic event. We return to Carmen's apartment. The tension leaves her face as her posterior hits the couch. She falls asleep.

HOW CAN I EVER THANK YOU?

December 15, 2011
Hello everyone,

So far so good, Carmen's first chemo treatment went well. She did not need a blood transfusion. The treatment lasted four hours. She was very anxious and hyperventilating and needed oxygen for the duration. That was very stressful for her but once she was home, she was able to relax and sleep. She won't lose her hair but it will thin out in three weeks or so. She has a small bed sore on her elbow (that has to be one strange sleeping position!). She's gained some weight – she's now 106 (not sure if that's with or without the Pamper). George and I were fired and so Lisa stayed with her last night.

It is crucial Carmen does not come in contact with anyone with a cold or other infection during her treatments (until end of January). Her immune system is very weak because of chemotherapy. If she gets a fever she will need to be hospitalized. So we have to be in prevention mode. The best way to prevent infections is to constantly wash your hands and wash them some more and ... again.

Keep the prayers coming folks!

Hugs all around. See you soon. Nicole XO

Help me live: Chapter 17 – "I don't know why I got cancer, and hearing your theory may add grave insult to injury."

- Did you smoke? Does it matter? The question makes you feel judged, defensive and guilty. Many people smoked longer and more than me and never got cancer. More important, many people who never smoked get lung cancer.
- A few people act as if you might be contagious or had done something to deserve the disease.
- A massage therapist suggested that I had brought on my own cancer through negative thoughts.
- There's always the undercurrent that if I had taken better care of myself, I would not be in this fix.
- "New age guilt" believes that cancer is "because of something". Sometimes we blame ourselves, "I must have gotten cancer because I somehow deserved it." It's all bull. Sometimes cancer just is and there's nothing spiritually related to why or where or who or when. It just is.
- Why did this happen? Why did the earthquake hit my house and not the neighbours? Why?
- We don't blame our pets when they get cancer. Why do we blame ourselves?
- You can help us live by leading us to the good places – and by staying there with us.

December 16, 2011
Hi everyone, just wanted to say if you phone my mom, she may not answer for a couple of days. She is very tired and trying to get as much rest as possible. She is doing well but sleeps a lot and does not have the energy to speak on the phone. She will get back to you when she is better. I slept there two nights; Martin is going to sleep there for the next two and then maybe George. We are taking it one day at a time. Thank you all for your support. Lisa

Joanne and her family leave for Jamaica for a week. Carmen had previously agreed to dog sit. She is too ill. George looks after Roxie. My sister adores it when the dog lies next to her on the couch. She resembles Candy, a dog Carmen had many years ago.

December 19, 2011

Well, I'm up, not too bad 4:30 A.M. I thought I would share my chemo experience of four hours. First my body turned into stone, could not breathe, very nervous. I was like a vegetable after for two or three days. I will not be taking the treatment on the 21st; I want to be fine for Christmas. Oh and by the way, if chemo is giving me anything beneficial I might reconsider, but for now it's bullshit. Like they said, it will not extend my life, then let God decide when he wants me. I love you all and can't wait to see you at Christmas. Carmen

Three months have passed since my sister's diagnosis. The distinct smell of chemo and medication are present throughout the entire apartment, predominately in my sister's bedroom. The toxins are released through perspiration and urination. My sister is told it can take six months to a year for her body to release these toxins. You smell it on my sister's clothes, her bed sheets, her mattress and even her couch.

Carmen verifies the water temperature in the bath – she flaps her hand in the water, it's nice and warm. She stands and lets her housecoat slip to the floor. She is naked. Her breasts are sagging; the contours of her ribs and her hip bones are visible; her skin is dry and flabby; she has little muscle tissue left, little fat. If this weight loss persists a black and white photo of my sister could easily belong in the Holocaust Memorial Museum in Washington DC.

This is the first time George is exposed to this – to a loved one, another human being, slowly dying of cancer and the effects that chemo brings.

George helps my sister into the bathtub. She grabs the bar for support as she steps in. A bar George installed a few weeks ago. She is lightweight; he holds her under her arms and gradually sits her in the tub. Carmen rests her left arm on the side of the tub to keep her PICC line out of the water. She does not wear the plastic cover recommended. It is uncomfortable and tight. Instead, George wraps a towel around her arm for protection. She soaks for a few minutes before he begins to wash her back. She has no strength to reach for her legs and her feet. He gently washes her entire body. She is tired; another day they will wash her hair.

George helps her out of the bathtub. Today she does not have the energy to dry herself, so he gently does and wraps her in her housecoat. They walk to the living room together; she lies down on her couch and reaches for the remote control and in minutes, she falls asleep.

George returns to clean the washroom, does another load of laundry and changes her bed.

> **December 21, 2011**
> Well, I went to bed at 8 P.M. and slept five hours straight, hard as a rock. I went for blood work yesterday for my other chemo treatment, which is today. I was in tears – I did not want to take anymore. I spoke with the pharmacist and she explained that today was a very small one, one hour tops. She said I could take my Ativan to calm me down. She said the chemo will shrink the tumor. Needless to say, my body is just like a bunch of nerves all tangled up. Let's hope it goes well. Did advise her I need to speak with the doctor for the big one. We will have to split it in two or they can keep me in the hospital for three days to recuperate. I love you all. Can't wait for the weekend with Denise, Sam, me and George. We will be going to an Auberge around the 28 before New Year's of course. I started drinking, what the hell. Afterwards, I will book quality time with the others. Nicole and I are taking the train this summer and going west. Love you all and to Julie, thank you so much for all you have done for me, Carmen
>
> **Later that day**
> Well, I have been meditating. I think I will snooze this one by. It will be an easy day. Now that is positive! Carmen

Barely recovered from her first chemo treatment, Carmen reluctantly agrees to attend the second. She is better prepared mentally. She takes her Ativan to calm her.

Once her treatment is done, we ask the nurse to look at her bedsore. She cleans it and gives us a few directives. We return home. Carmen sleeps.

Within days, the bedsore is infected. George brings her to emergency. Antibiotics are administered by intravenous. She is required to come to the hospital three times daily for seven days for her medication. They prefer she stays at home, given her reduced immunity as a result of chemo. A hospital is not the place to be. Most are challenged with superbugs; the likes of C difficile and MRSA. Carmen could easily acquire these drug resistant infections and other bacteria. The daily appointments in addition to the side effects of chemo are demanding and difficult on my sister. She needs to dress properly for the cold winter, the travel time, the waiting. It does not give her enough time to rest and recover from her treatments. She has little energy. She is suffering. We don't know what to think, what to expect. Is this reasonable?

You rely on the system; you rely on the health care team and the experts. As I watch my sister suffer, I secretly hope she will not take chemo again. Many patients die from the effects of chemo and not their cancer. I respect my sister's decision. She is fighting to live. I would probably do the same.

We gather at my place for Christmas. David, Karen and their children come up from Kitchener; Mom and Tim from the Niagara region. The entire family is in Ottawa except for Denise. She and her children spend their traditional Christmas in Saint-Sauveur. Carmen fights to be with us at Christmas. She has a constant struggle with fatigue, nausea, other side effects, and the pain in her foot, leg and sitting bones. She spends the night lying on my sofa surrounded by family watching her sleep.

Carmen and George leave early that evening. We continue our celebration. Karen returns to the room crying. She sits next to Joanne. Clueless, I ask, "What's going on? What happened?"

"What do you mean what happened?" says Joanne, "It's Carmen!"

Karen last saw my sister at their annual "Miller July 1st weekend." You become blind and accustomed to your surroundings. I realize I no longer see Carmen's gradual decline.

Our nephew, Adam, Denise's son, comes down between Christmas and New Year's Eve. He wants to see Carmen. He wants her to meet his son, Leo, who is six weeks old. After one of her daily appointments at the hospital, Carmen comes over for a visit. She sits on the living room sofa next to Mom. She finds the baby beautiful. She is too weak to take him. Struggling with this awful fatigue, she barely stayed ten minutes. George starts the car;

it's still warm. In the meantime, Carmen sits as we slip on her boots. "Help me to the car, Adam." She holds onto him as they walk. She needs to sleep.

Adam and his life partner, Sophie are shocked to see how much Carmen has deteriorated in the last two months. When Adam returns home, he telephones his mother, "You better go see her quickly. She's dying. I don't think she has much more time to live."

December 31, 2011
Good morning everyone,

Yep, it's 2:06 A.M., can't sleep – my feet are sooo swollen they keep me awake. I have been debating for a few days if I will continue chemo. I have made the decision I will not be taking it any more. I decided to let nature take its course. The two treatments I received have made me very sick and did not give me a quality life. I will meet with the oncologist on the fourth and tell him. He can tell me who I see if I am sick, my family doctor or them, and take that friggin PICC line off my arm so I can take a 20-minute bath. I was very happy to see everybody at Christmas. It was too bad I had caught the bacteria and had to go to the hospital three times a day, and then did not want to miss visiting you. So that really burnt the candles at both ends. Yesterday I was starting to get stronger. I guess I needed the rest. Well, I want to wish you all a Happy New Year, and I know in a few weeks I will get my legs back and then I shall start visiting. One week at Mom's and one week at David's (I guess you will have to give me your bed, David hihi). Then Denise and cottage again with my two angels with spouse.

Love you all. Happy New Year. Carmen

Roger and I spend a quiet New Year's Eve together at home. We had not made any plans for celebration. I cry and sip my champagne, "My sister is not dead but I feel I have already lost her."

I feel helpless. I don't know what is "normal" anymore. I have lost all interest in socializing and entertaining. It is too much effort. It will be like this for a year.

★ ★ ★

At times, Carmen thinks of moving into a seniors' residence or a type of palliative care centre where she could be taken care of. It would give the family a break and she would have care 24 hours a day. When we discuss it, we tell her, "Later, wait until we can no longer care for you, wait until you need medical attention."

"It's expensive. You will have to choose between your apartment and the residence. What's your preference?" I ask.

"No. I don't want to let go of my apartment."

"You'll be more comfortable here sis, especially in the summer time. You will be able to sit outside, catch a few sun rays and hang out with your friends on the swing, like you used to."

January 4, 2012
Hi Family,

Just wanted to give you an update. Today was my mom's appointment with her oncologist. She told him she did not want to go on with chemo. She wants to try without for a bit and see if her quality of life will improve. He was very nice and sympathetic. He agreed to take her PICC line out, and in less than a week, she will be able to take a FULL BATH and she is sooo excited. She is cutting down the cortisone, which is what is making her face swollen; she is now down to a half, one a day for a week and then she's done. The doctor says it will take about one month for the swelling to go down.

He will still be the one to follow her, even if she is not doing chemo. He wants to see her on March 21st for a follow up, and to know if she would like to continue with chemo. She will make that decision later in time. Now her main goal is to spend time with her friends and family. I can now say she will be able to rest. Knowing she had to do chemo was an enormous stress on her and a lot of work.

Mom, I love you and I am very proud of you for being so strong. And thanks to all of you for being such a good family and friends. Lisa

Our lives have changed since September 17, 2011. Lisa lost the baby, only to become pregnant again three months later. Her due date is September 17, 2012. Twelve months to the day Carmen was initially hospitalized for her cancer. My grandmother used to say, "Death brings a life." It explains why we find obituaries next to birth announcements in newspapers.

George picks up my sister's mail. He keeps the envelope from an insurance company for me and delivers the rest to my sister. It's another insurance form for a physician to sign. I will contact them tomorrow. Today we bring Carmen to see her family physician. She needs to renew a prescription. They cannot do it by phone. He wants to see her.

His new office in Gatineau is adjacent to a pharmacy and close to the hospital. We temporarily park in the handicap parking. We help Carmen out of the car and sit her on her walker. I push her through the snow and up the icy sidewalk while George holds the doors open. We leave the oxygen tank in the car. My sister feels strong enough to do without for this short visit. We wheel her to the reception; the employee informs us they have a wheelchair and complains because we have not removed our boots and snow is on the floor. The wheelchair is at the back of the room. I collect it and we transfer Carmen from her walker to the chair. The receptionist, still complaining about the floor, walks out with a mop. She is upset, this is chaos for her. The physician overhears. He greets my sister, grabs the wheelchair by the handles and wheels my sister into his office. His non-verbal cues suggest we don't know what we are doing. George takes the mop from the receptionist and starts cleaning the floor. She returns to her desk, still complaining and giving orders. George doesn't acknowledge her commands. He simply rolls his eyes in disgust.

I remove my boots and slide on a pair of blue plastic slippers. Reflecting on the drama, I'm thinking *what a character*. She can easily get under your skin. As we wait for Carmen, another patient arrives. He automatically removes his boots.

The physician is surprised Carmen is discontinuing chemotherapy, "It can prolong your life!" She's heard these words before. Barely in his office a few minutes, he hands her the new prescription and brings her to the waiting room. As we leave, Carmen informs us that Janet, the receptionist, is the physician's wife. "She was a clerk with the federal government. She quit her job to work with her husband."

The next day I'm back, facing Janet (with a new pair of plastic slippers). I need a copy of Carmen's last chest X-ray for the insurance company. It seems complicated, but she finally agrees to send me a report by email. The physician walks over and joins our conversation.

"When do we know it's time to bring my sister to a palliative care centre?" I ask.

"Does she have homecare?"

"No. She had a nurse come in weekly to clean her PICC line."

"She can still get around."

"But barely," I correct him. "You saw her yesterday. That was one of her better days. They gave her one year. How do we know when it's time?"

"Once she has palliative care at home, by my experience, it's about six months."

My eyes are watery, "And who decides on homecare? Is it the family?"

"No. Her medical team will make that decision. Once she can no longer get out, they will provide homecare. The physician will visit her at home. She may spend her last few months in a palliative care centre."

I'm holding back the tears. As I leave I hear, "Bon courage." I know it's genuine. I feel their compassion.

The next day Janet sends me the documentation by email. I forward the information to the insurance company. They want proof Carmen did not have lung cancer before purchasing the car loan insurance. I contact the representative to discuss the next steps. He informs me of another form to be completed by the oncologist on my sister's status.

"Not another form for the oncologist to sign!" I explain, "You know. They don't want to complete these forms. The last time it cost my sister $150. I don't understand. What else do you need?"

"The outcome of her chemo treatments; it's our policy."

"The oncologist does not have that information. My sister is scheduled for a CT Scan early next month and the results won't be in for your deadline. In Quebec, it takes four weeks to get results of a biopsy." I go on, "My sister is dying. Her cancer is at stage IV. Regardless that the chemo treatments have reduced the size of her tumours, she will never go back to work; not to her old position or any other. She is too weak. She can't get around. She has terminal cancer. She has one year to live. She is told continuously that these treatments will not prolong her life or cure her cancer. They are administered for a better quality of life, which is very poor."

He is quiet. I proceed, "You know, we have a shortage of oncologists. Their time is better spent treating patients." I pause and add, "Completing these forms adds stress to a cancer patient. They don't need to worry about their financial affairs. It's a simple form to us but it is stressful for them. Simple and regular things are overwhelming to them."

"I understand. I'll delay the request until your sister meets with her oncologist next and you can phone me with the results; no additional forms will be sent. It will be the last."

I thanked him. He kept his word.

David makes it a priority to spend time with Carmen. He does so once a month. He leaves Kitchener late morning, a five-hour drive, has dinner with our sister, they watch a movie together and talk. He returns home early the next morning, leaving before rush hour. Carmen loves her younger brother. She loves their brief visits together. She is grateful he makes time for her.

On occasion, George will stay but he usually doesn't. He gives them privacy. We all respect each other's time with Carmen.

I'm at Chapters Indigo again, this time outside the self-help section. I can't decide which book my sister would prefer so I buy the two. *Twinkle Twinkle Little Star* and *All the Ways I love You*. Two baby books; the kind where you record your voice while reading the story.

"A souvenir you can leave your grandchild," I say when I see her next.

She smiles with gratitude. She records her voice a few times. She's still not satisfied. She is tired. She will finalize it later.

Carmen wants to celebrate George's birthday. She makes reservations at the restaurant for friends and family who can attend. The restaurant is spacious and our table is back at the far end. Carmen manages to walk with the pain shooting up her leg. She did not want us to bring the walker. It took all her energy to make it to the table. Her face is swollen from the medication. She is fighting to stay longer, her sitting bones ache. The wooden chairs add to her discomfort.

It's time to leave. I warm up the car and wait in the lobby of the restaurant. Carmen arrives, sitting in a chair carried by James and Martin, just like a goddess high in the air. George is behind, holding the portable oxygen tank.

February 18, 2012
Hi everyone. Got a call from Jennifer, told me Aunt Pierrette's husband died today. I think it was around six. Carmen

Pierrette, my father's sister, remarried years ago. Her second husband had lung cancer. He had been suffering and was in palliative care for many months before passing away.

"He's dead! He was at stage III and I'm at stage IV!" I can't describe Carmen's facial expression. I respond, "He probably had a different type of lung cancer. He's been in palliative care for a while. You are at home. "

A friend, a director of a palliative care centre, shares with me that medical intervention disrupts a patient's emotional and spiritual progress. They seem to lose control of their life, as if it is given to the medical team during treatments. They take control of their own life once the treatments cease.

I can see it with Carmen. It is a roller coaster ride. When she is subjected to treatment; she is fighting for her life. All her concentration is on chemo. Her mental state is different. She is frightened. When she chooses to let nature take its course, her transformation, her journey is underway. She is more reflective, her anger and impatience diminishes, and she is more forgiving and accepting, more at peace. She is in the present. She is preparing to enter a new world.

"Mentally, you can easily let yourself go. When you are this sick, it's easy to let yourself die." I listen to my sister as I'm massaging her legs.

Carmen slides the pulse oximeter on her index finger. She waits a few seconds for the reading. Her oxygen saturation is at 98 and so is her pulse. She removes it and returns it to the coffee table.

"If I did not have so much help, if George had not taken care of me, I would be dead," she continues. "I was so tired; I could not get out of bed; I could not lift my body off the toilet even with the support bars; George had to lift and carry me. I felt like I had been hit by a truck. My body ached everywhere. I wanted to let myself go, let myself die. It would have been easy you know." After a brief pause she adds, "I regret taking chemo."

I feel little fat or muscle tissue on her legs. The body cream is quickly absorbed with every stroke. Her skin is dry, another side effect of chemo and the medication.

"I hear you, sis. You were so sick at Christmas. I can't believe what you are going through. Chemo is hard. Thank God we have George."

I wipe my hands on the towel. She sprints to the washroom with her new walk – small rapid steps with both feet dragging. She returns with a disgusted look.

"What is it?" I ask.

"I can't stand that chemo. I smell it when I urinate."

★ ★ ★

Lisa's pregnancy is at risk. Due to the nature of her work, her obstetrician suggests a three-day work week instead of five. She needs more rest.

"If my back and stomach aches persist, my physician recommends a full-time medical leave until the baby is born," shares Lisa.

She sits close to her mother on the couch.

"You do as she says, Lisa."

Gently resting her head on Lisa's tummy, Carmen speaks to her grandchild.

"The baby can hear me, you know."

A CONSTANT BATTLE

"I have cancer, stage IV, I'm dying. Don't you understand?" she repeats with a bitter voice. George continues to be in denial. It's the only way he can live through this. He relies on his faith. He believes in miracles. He cares for her. They soon depart for the hospital for another medical consultation. It's now six months post my sister's diagnosis.

March 21, 2012
Hi folks,

Here is an update. I went to see my oncologist and he told me my tumor had shrunk 60%. That's a BIG number! I was very happy to hear the news. Keep your prayers going, don't quit, I am sure God has heard you. Thanks everyone for caring. Love you Carmen

What a boost! She feels better psychologically and physically. She does not cough like she used to.

That same week, we celebrate Martin's birthday. He invites a few friends and his aunts to the restaurant. We have early reservations; Carmen does not have the stamina for late evenings. She's proud of her "beluga," a nickname she gave her son a few years back.

April 7, 2012
Any more chapters left on help me live??? I started waking up every morning at 4 A.M. I used to wake up and think, when is my day coming? Not looking forward to it. But now the cancer shrank and now the question is, is it growing back? I guess it's a no win situation. I am doing better, but I hate having to feel dependent on everybody. Maybe it's the hardest part, that I am limited. Please keep your prayers going. I have deleted Lisa on this email as I do not want to put stress on her. She has to have a nice

> pregnancy. Well anyway, I just thought I would share this with you, as sometimes we wonder what a cancer patient feels. Love you all and thanks for everything.

Moments later, our nephew Patrick, Denise's eldest, sends us a refreshing email about his ten-year-old son.

> Hi, Jonathan scored the winning goal in the first hockey game of the tournament this morning. His team, the Canadians, tied the game with 12 seconds remaining on the clock. He was picked by the coach for his first shootout attempt. He's very happy. I think he'll remember this one for a very long time.
>
> Enjoy the short video.

★ ★ ★

I try to summarize another book for Carmen's 4 A.M. readings. This one was sent to me by Louise, Carmen's friend. It's a deep and heavy read and difficult to summarize. I send my sister a few summaries but it does not have the same effect. It's too complex. The only thing my sister retains is that the body is a "rented domicile"[9].

I can't answer the house phone, my hands are full. I let it go to the answering machine. Seconds later I hear my cell phone ring from a distance. Then the house phone rings again. I know it's my sister. Carmen describes to me her latest meeting with the oncologist. She asked him, "If my tumour shrank by 60%, can my cancer be at stage II?"

He pats her shoulder gently and replies, "No. Your cancer will always remain at stage IV."

I hear silence on the phone, then I listen to her cry. I wait until she's done.

"I guess the pat on the shoulder didn't help things any." She laughs at my reply.

---

[9] Levine, Stephen. *Who Dies? An investigation of Conscious Living and Conscious Dying.* New York: Doubleday, 1982. Print.

Another yo-yo episode of hope, denial and reality; every one becomes more difficult. Dr. Jones does not tell her how long she has to live, "It's God's decision."

April 12, 2012
Your opinion please. I added a few things to the letter. Have a nice trip, will miss you sis. Carmen

My reply
That's a beautiful thank you letter, sis. George will love it. No doubt this will bring tears to his eyes. I knew you could find it in you to write such a heartwarming letter. Now … if we could only work on your snapping turtle reflex!

See you Monday. Have a good weekend. Love you. Nicole

In her letter, she thanks George and loves him for all he has done for her, how her children have always regarded him as their father, how he needs to continue to be part of their lives and of course, his obligations as the only "Pappy". She directs him to spoil and love their grandchild for both of them.

★ ★ ★

My sister receives a statement from her lawyer. She sends another payment; she can't afford to pay the total. Her chest tightens. She wonders when the trial will be.

Roger knows the file well. He met with Carmen and her lawyer a year ago to review the evidence. It is clearly an injustice. He recommends trying to find a resolution without going through the legal system. To do this, Carmen would have to share her defense with the new board of the cooperative. It's a risk she is willing to take. She gives him full responsibility. They don't inform her lawyer.

Roger offers his assistance to the chair and board of the cooperative. They need expertise and coaching. The financial institution forced the board to relinquish all responsibilities and in turn, gave a third party a management agreement.

Roger attends the cooperative's annual general meeting. A history of bad blood among the members contributes to their problems. Roger introduces himself and explains how he can assist the board. The membership accepts. He begins coaching the board shortly after.

> **April 26, 2012 from Carmen to me**
> I went to bed at 9 P.M. and woke up at 1:30 A.M. I said I am not getting up, but had a headache and just sat in bed; took the glass of water and of course it fell in my bottle of Tylenol. They were all wet and I had to pick up the mess. I went back to bed, slept on and off. I'm going for a test today and I have all these ideas in my head, where has my positiveness gone to? I wonder why I bother taking all these tests, it won't change anything. I wonder if the cancer grew. I'm crying because I'm scared I won't make it for Lisa in September. I feel as if my body is trying to tell me to let go. Maybe I should see somebody to talk to from the Cancer Society. Anyway I will be off this morning for another scan and I might go see my "Pivot" nurse. I will call you when I get back. Love your bosom, Carmen.

That moment I forward the email to Denise, David and Joanne.

> Hi siblings,
> I thought I would share with you, in confidence, how your sister is feeling. I could tell something was up – she's been odd these past few days. It's like her mind is continuously fighting with her body.
>
> I'm past my competence level on this one. I'll try to find a support group to help me help her. I can see how difficult it is for someone who is ill, suffering physically and mentally, to actually go out for counselling or schedule appointments at home. You never know how you are going to feel or what energy level you will have on a given day. It takes her days to recuperate from a medical appointment.
>
> She's at the hospital this morning for a scan. She just found out it will take her most of the day. She was injected with the contrast

liquid at 10 A.M.; the nuclear scan is scheduled for 1 P.M. She will be in the scanner for 45 minutes. No doubt she will be very tired. This is a long day for her. I tried to encourage her to see her nurse coordinator, since she's at the hospital, to inquire on the type of counselling available. She is somewhat resistant – I can understand. I will keep you posted. Talk to you soon, Nicole

My reply to Carmen
I hear you bosom sis. I've been thinking ... we need help for this!

Some ideas ...

1. Social worker/spiritual care provider from the hospital (oncology dept.) may be able to help. Do you want me to call?
2. *Maison Mathieu Froment-Savoie*. They may offer help at home. I left a message for them to call me back re: what's available for patients and caregivers.
3. Check this website - it looks very informative. You can ask questions online to professionals plus so much more. www.virtualhospice.ca

I want to help you. We talk and think together, OK?
Love you, your bosom sister.

We briefly discuss it later that day. She needs to rest. She will look at the website another time. Carmen communicates best in the morning when she is more energetic, when she is ready. To have such discussions at home does not lend itself naturally; the phone rings constantly, the television is on and the volume is high, neighbours drop in and she sleeps on the couch on and off.

May 1, 2011
PLEASE NOTE THIS EMAIL WAS NOT SENT TO LISA. I DO NOT WANT TO WORRY HER. Last week I was not feeling too well MENTALLY, physically I'm the same. Nicole found me a cancer site and I wrote to them, so I thought I would share their reply with you. Scroll down, love you all. Carmen

Ask a Professional: Inbox
Welcome Tinour!

[Interesting my sister chose to identify herself as "Tinour," French slang for "little bear," a nickname given to her by our father. When she was young and angry, she would have the temperament of a little bear. She was upset when anyone else used the nickname. Only Dad could call her Tinour.]

Your question: I have stage IV cancer in both lungs. I had radio and chemo. Chemo was making me very sick, I looked and felt like I was dying so I quit everything. I try to be very strong but sometimes I can't stop crying. I am not scared of dying but I don't want to let go. My cancer had shrunk 60% but even if it grew back a bit, I cannot take chemo. I have lost interest in everything. I am a prisoner in my house. If I go out, it takes me days to recover and I feel I cannot burden my family with my thoughts, they already have a hard time dealing with this. What can I do to help me deal with this?

Hello Tinour,

We are sorry to hear about your diagnosis of lung cancer and difficulty with chemotherapy. We feel privileged that you have taken the time to share your experience, thoughts and feelings with us. This takes courage and strength. In your short message you have conveyed so many of the struggles, fears, feelings of loss, loneliness, isolation, sadness, and concern for family. These are common amongst those living with advanced cancer and limited time. While it may be of small comfort, sometimes it is reassuring to know that you are not alone and that what you are experiencing is natural or similar to that of others.

Our personal and professional experience affirms that human beings are amazingly resilient. In the face of difficulty and stress, we can learn, adapt and work our way through what is put in front of us. Crying is part of this work … it is a natural reflection of the losses (loss of health, loss of usual activities, loss of life) and sadness that we are experiencing. It is part of acknowledging these losses, trying to come to terms with them and moving forward. Crying is not about being "less strong".

Stopping treatment is a tough decision; and again demonstrates your personal strength and courage in being able to do so. Stopping treatment is not about "giving up" but rather about opening yourself to what is currently being experienced and figuring out how best to live it. Terminating cancer-focused treatment creates a space in life to focus on what is most important to you … how you want to spend the time remaining. We encourage you to think about what are the life goals or things that are most important for you to do. The *Topics* article written by our clinical team address a wide range of subjects: under "Emotional and Spiritual Health" that you may find beneficial.

Stopping cancer-focused treatment also opens the opportunity to choose palliative care as an alternate approach. We encourage you to explore with your cancer care team (doctors and nurses) how to be referred or connected to hospice palliative care services in your area.

We respect your concern for your family and your wish not to "burden them". This is also a common concern of those living with serious illness. However, during this time of living with limited energy, it sometimes takes a lot of energy to keep people away or protect them. While they are perhaps having trouble coming to terms with the realities of your illness, they may also want to help but feel helpless and unsure about how to do so. Being open and honest with each other is often "freeing" for everyone (in other words, it's like talking about the "elephant in the room"). Family members often try to protect each other; while sharing the same thoughts, concerns and questions. Perhaps there is an opportunity for you to come together, to talk and support each other. Each person/family is unique, therefore the ways you communicate with each other will depend on what "fits" for you, but we encourage you to do so if possible. A place to start, might be sharing what is on your mind, giving them permission to do the same. Another place to start, might be asking if they would like to help and identifying practical ways for them to do so.

Living with uncertainty and limited time can be stressful and overwhelming. Breaking it down into small chunks may be useful ... worrying about today and what you would like or need to do. Accepting and planning for help around your home, grocery shopping/errands, or with your personal care, may help you to conserve energy for what you really want to do.

We commend you for being able to share your experience and reach out for help. In caring for individuals living with serious illness, those who are able to express their thoughts, concerns and questions as well as seek out information and assistance, often tell us that this makes a big difference in their ability to cope.

A couple of suggestions of places to start to inquire about support services in your area. Often hospice palliative care and Cancer Society offices have staff and/or specially trained volunteers who offer a "listening ear," emotional/spiritual support and practical assistance. If these offices do not provide the services you are looking for, hopefully they can connect you to other local resources. These offices may also be able to connect you to home care services if needed.

We hope this is helpful.

★ ★ ★

Carmen wakes to the sound of the door opening. Another interrupted snooze on the couch. She lifts her head from the cushion, it's Lisa. She is happy to see her.

"Hi Mom. I brought you a chicken casserole. I just made it. It's still warm."

Lisa is now on full-time medical leave. The baby is growing.

She prepares a serving for her mother and she does as she is told. She sits on the couch next to her. Carmen rubs her daughter's tummy and talks to her grandson. It becomes common practice. My sister is proud of her daughter and happy for her.

"You and James will be great parents."

> **May 4, 2012**
> I don't know if I did something or said something yesterday, but I found you very frustrated just talking with me. Please let me know what I did. It is better to get it off your chest than to keep it bottled inside. If you tell me, I will try not to do it again. Sorry, Carmen.

Carmen sent me this email along with a picture of me, her and Denise probably taken by Joanne a few years ago en route to Sudbury to visit Dad's grave.

I feel sick to my stomach when I read this email. I do not know what to say. I always thought Carmen had difficulty communicating and here the shoe fits on my foot. How do I reply to this? I have my days. I'm tired of hearing my phone ring. We speak many times daily; the same conversations. It seems worse when I tell her I'm busy. I'm having a tough time studying for my Spanish exams and my Sommelier program. How can I tell her to stop calling so often? My problems are nothing compared to hers. I wish others would pick up some slack.

I phone her as I'm having my cup of coffee. Jokingly I say, "Can I not have my moments? Am I no longer entitled to PMS?" We carry on our conversation and agree to send each other five things we are grateful for in our lives. This becomes our daily task.

> **May 4, 2012**
> Hi sis,
>
> Can't use the same every day, love you.
>
> Gratitude, thankfulness, gratefulness, or appreciation is a feeling, emotion or attitude in acknowledgement of a benefit that one has received or will receive. With the advent of the positive

psychology movement, gratitude has become a mainstream focus of psychological research.

I am grateful to have today.
I am grateful I have two wonderful children plus a grandson coming soon.
I am grateful I have a bosom sister who cares very much for me even if she snaps at me.
I am grateful Roger is taking care of my shit in the coop.
I am grateful I have a roof over my head.
Carmen

My reply
Today ... or should I say yesterday ...

I'm grateful I have a bosom sister Carmen.
I'm grateful I can physically practice yoga. I feel so good afterwards.
I'm grateful for the fragrance of flowers.
I'm grateful for the sunshine and its effect on my mood.
I'm grateful my sister has a good sense of humour.

I came in too late last night to send my email!
Nicole

May 5, 2012
I guess I was playing by myself, did the wine take over????
I am grateful my son comes on Saturday morning - gives us quality time.
I am grateful my children call me everyday.
I am grateful it is sunny outside, it lifts my spirits.
I am grateful I am not going downhill with my sickness.
I am grateful we have a close knit family.
Carmen

My reply
I'm grateful I was not hurt with my motorcycle accident.
I'm grateful my husband is understanding.
I'm grateful to hear the birds sing and the bees buzz.
I'm grateful for the warm weather.
I'm grateful I can relax at home.
Nicole

May 6, 2012
I am grateful I was able to sit outside a few hours on the swing.
I am grateful my sister lends me her husband for my only outing.
I am grateful George has a new activity, his bike.
I am grateful Lisa put the phone on her tummy and I talk to my grandchild.
I am grateful Julie came to visit me today even if she looks very tired.
Carmen

My reply
I am grateful I'm not pregnant (thanks for the tip).
I am grateful Martin took the time to visit me and fix my motorcycle (looks like new).
I am grateful for my washer and dryer and the smell of my clean clothes.
I am grateful my husband plays with my sister.
I am grateful for my property (although it's a lot of work).
Nicole

As I'm speaking to Carmen on the phone, I hear a beep. She puts me on hold to answer her other line. "It's Brigitte."

"Who's Brigitte?" I ask.

"She's a neighbour. We have known each other for years. I hired her to clean my apartment."

"We can do that for you, sis. You don't need to pay someone."

Silence, seconds later I hear her crying, "I don't want to burden anyone. I want to do things myself…"

It took me a quick second to reply, "You're right. My cleaning lady comes in bi-weekly. You'll feel better if you have someone come in as well."

"I want a good spring cleaning. George can't do everything. He already does so much," she continues to cry.

"You're right, sis. It's a good idea."

May 7, 2012
I am grateful my sister came to visit even if I slept in her face.
I am grateful I was able to go out with my sister for pogo and fries.
I am grateful it was a beautiful day.
I am grateful my sister brought her dog because I love animals.
I am grateful I have a computer to send this to my bosom.
Carmen

My reply
I'm grateful for the feel of clean, crisp linen on my bed.
I'm grateful I have a bed and a roof over my head.
I'm grateful for the big, thick worms I find in my lawn. It means it's healthy.
I'm grateful my sister-in-law invites us for dominos and dinner.
I'm grateful my husband is a good cook.
Nicole

May 8, 2012
I'm grateful I have a couch to sleep on.
I'm grateful for snoozzzzzzzzzzz.
I am grateful people I don't know are praying for me.
I am grateful God helps me when I have bad thoughts about giving up.
I am grateful my bosom sister's husband takes care of me.
Carmen

My reply
I'm grateful it's raining today because our sprinkler system needs repair and the lawn seeds need water.
I'm grateful I can smell the clean, crisp air after a rainfall.

I'm grateful my sister shares her journey with me.
I'm grateful I'm currently not working.
I'm grateful for my coffee in the morning.
I'm grateful we have a three-day break on grateful things!
Nicole

I don't recall why we took a break, but we never returned to the task of our five grateful things.

★ ★ ★

We all try in our own ways to help Carmen as best we can. Joanne sends her an email.

> ... in case you wake up in the middle of the night and needed something to read ... I want you to know I love you very much and only want the best for you. Sometimes it's hard for me to find the right things to say when I don't know what to say. Sometimes listening feels like it's just not enough. I wish I could take this illness away and make things better but I can't. Nobody can ... I understand you when you feel like you are climbing up a ladder and then get knocked down to the bottom after hearing not so good news ... my wish for you ... is for you to be at peace with this disease and for you to enjoy the time we have left together. I think of the future and I see you at Lisa's baby shower having fun. I see you at David's cottage enjoying the family reunion and the birthday celebrations. I see you on your birthday ... probably at the casino! I see you in the delivery room with Lisa (and Nicole passed out on the floor!). I see you rocking Lucas to sleep. I see you celebrating Christmas ... because we have to redo last year's Christmas ... you were too sick. I see you singing lullabies to Lucas like the ones Dad used to sing to us. I see you at peace and starting your new journey.
>
> In one of Nicole's email messages ... the quote ... *A friend told me I was wrapped in her love and prayers* - I never forgot those words. I love that statement. You, Carmen, are wrapped in my love and

prayers. Love you so very much,
Joanne

Carmen's reply
Thank you so much, I thought I had no more tear drops but I guess I do but made it last for five minutes. I love you a lot and I know we are all helpless, but everything will work fine one day at a time. Love you lots, sis.

I receive a phone call from Carmen. She is upset with Lisa and starts crying on the phone. A bout like no other, worse than the one she had with me at the hospital. She is heartbroken. Lisa is having a birthday party and has not invited her mother.

"But she's spending her birthday with you and the family on Thursday. This is a party with her friends." I try to console her.

"Yes, but she always invited me before. I know her friends. I'm too sick to stay for long but I would try to go. This is the last birthday I can spend with her." And she continues to cry. She puts down the receiver. I hear her blowing her nose. She returns. I tell her, "Well, you know how selfish kids are."

Denise is with her. She tells me Carmen has been crying throughout the day. She has never seen her this way. George and I have. The emotions are powerful; people are tender but Carmen is raw.

I text Lisa, "Whatever the reason … just invite your mom." She replies, "Yes. It's so complicated."

Sometimes you just can't think straight. Hormonal changes or a pregnancy brain may play a part. The following week Lisa cancels the party with her friends and celebrates her birthday with her family as planned.

We learn that it's OK to say or do the wrong thing. People forgive. I witnessed many occasions where my sister demonstrated amazing strength and serenity under demanding circumstances. I try to do the same.

★ ★ ★

I meet a few girlfriends for dinner. The conversation turns to my sister. Eventually they share their common opinion that the medical team should not disclose how long a terminally ill patient has to live.

Helen shares her experience with cancer, and Theresa, her sister-in-law's. I'm not sure if they differentiate between curing and palliative. I wonder if people faced with terminal illness want honesty. Is anyone ever ready for such awful news? Would you want to know your prognosis? How else do we acknowledge it's real? Perhaps it's part of our transformation, our journey to the next world.

The prognosis may help the patient and family prepare for death. It may help them prioritize the time they have remaining. It gives them the opportunity to share how much they love each other. To get there, we need to stop pretending. Everyone has to acknowledge the elephant in the room. Dying is a process.

It's a complex subject with many different views. I don't have the heart to explain mine when I don't fully comprehend it myself. If I try, I may cry. I'm in another world.

★ ★ ★

Lisa agrees to Carmen attending the birth of her first born. "Not a problem. Invite whoever you want and as many as you want," responds her obstetrician.

Carmen has made up her mind. I am to attend with her, given her condition, in case she needs help. If I'm to replace her as the grandmother, I need to play the role. I have no choice. I let it go, thinking it probably won't happen; she will be too sick to observe the birth.

★ ★ ★

Sitting next to her on the couch, I listen to my sister cry as I hold her in my arms. She turns and looks at me with her big, brown, sad and teary eyes, "How are you going to live without your bosom sister?"

Our watery eyes meet but I have no words.

I think of her life, how much she struggled through so much, so many times. I think of how much she has given. She is proud of her two children. As a single mother on a low income, she assumed both roles and did it well. The children's father was absent from the very beginning and contributed very little financially or otherwise to his children's welfare. The little Carmen had, she shared with family and friends in need.

I wish I could tell her everything is going to be all right.

June 18, 2012

Nine months post my sister's diagnosis.

Carmen sends me a link to the Canadian Virtual Hospice on finding peace at the end-of-life. The topics range from various emotions, helping you find peace, connecting with others. I'm pleased to see she is reading on the subject.

It's the July 1st weekend – Miller time, David's annual family gathering.

Anne, Lisa's close friend, is coming to the party. Martin tells David he wants to bring her as his date. David phones me, "We don't bring friends. We don't even have enough room for the family. I can't tell Karen, she'll freak out!"

"I know what you're saying. Just tell Karen it's his new girlfriend. Don't muck this up, we are trying to match them up together."

Martin eventually breaks up with his girlfriend (to Carmen's chagrin. I should say happiness, really). Now single, he and Anne drive to David's cottage together.

Early morning on the day of our departure, Roger and I drive to Carmen's and load up the rented 25 foot RV with all the oxygen cylinders, the oxygen concentrator (her R2D2 as Carmen's calls it), cases of beer and luggage. The RV is parked at the front entrance of her building. Neighbours come to inspect. Carmen is lying on the bed. She is happy and looking forward to the trip. George securely ties the oxygen cylinder in the centre of the RV. Carmen can walk to the table, the bed and the washroom.

Roger drives, George is in the passenger seat and I stay at the back with Carmen. She takes her morphine and spends most of the trip in bed. She has no seatbelt but at this point, it doesn't matter. It's the only way we can bring her to the party. It is impossible for her to sit in a car that long.

We take the scenic route through the Algonquin Provincial Park to avoid major highways. We neglect to check off "avoid off road" on the GPS. Roger takes a dirt road as per the directions; Carmen is bouncing all over the bed with every bump. "Are we lost? Do you guys know what you are doing?"

It's clear after 15 minutes we are not on the right road but you don't turn around a 25 foot RV just anywhere. "Is this the right road? Are we lost?" repeats Carmen.

We come to a house and the men ask for directions. A slight detour and we are back on the main highway.

We stop at Casino Rama en route. Roger finds a wheelchair and the two of them go in to try their luck while George and I prepare a healthy salad in the camper. They did not win; apparently, George and I were too close to the facility, we brought them bad luck. Although Carmen found it uncomfortable and long, it was the perfect means of travel in her condition.

We are 36 people this year; three can't attend the reunion. David's cottage is full; his yard is covered with tents and cars are parked everywhere.

That weekend we pre-celebrated Roger and Carmen's 60th birthdays. Carmen slept in the cottage. George, Roger and I stayed in the RV. Between the party, the noisy air conditioning unit and everyone's snoring, we did not sleep all weekend.

Later in the week, with the help of Anne, Carmen holds a baby shower for Lisa. It is a full day for her. She is determined to find the strength. She wants something special for her beautiful daughter. She succeeds.

July 9, 2012
Hi sis,

> Go on this site - this is the treatment I am receiving: Lung cancer and Malignant pleural mesothelioma.

The waiting room is full, practically every seat is taken. Carmen is in a wheelchair, I'm sitting and George is standing. We are waiting for Carmen's number to appear on the screen. The oncology department has a new automated system and the wait is incredible. People are tolerant given that it is their second day in operation. It's clearly not working; people are waiting hours before their treatment. The patients are sick; any additional delay is difficult for them. Peter, disabled and in a wheelchair, works diligently to help patients in the confusion. He's a new volunteer with a beautiful smile and a great sense of humour.

Two other volunteers make their rounds, offering beverages and a light lunch to patients. Carmen eats a ham sandwich on white bread. She leaves the crust behind. She holds on to her juice.

A small two-seater sofa becomes available. We give it to Carmen so she may lie down in a fetus position and rest. Every seat is taken. The place is busy.

The man sitting next to me is proud to share that his daughter is the architect who designed this room, the glass wall and ceiling including the special ornaments.

He stops his explanation when a young woman in tears arrives with her father into the waiting room. The man, in a wheelchair, appears to be in his 60s. He is calm. Peter wheels his way over to help her. We listen to their conversation.

"There is nothing they can do for him. The doctor said they did all they could," she cries.

Her father wiggles in his wheelchair and says something in a foreign language. Her hand on her father's shoulder, she tells the volunteer, "My father doesn't like it when I cry."

Every single one of us in this room can relate to this situation, to their pain.

My neighbour looks at my sister, "Family makes it difficult. It's the worst part." She nods in agreement.

Carmen's number is finally posted. We make our way to the room. She prefers I attend with her. "George does not ask the right questions, he's in denial."

We enter the room and wait for the physician to arrive. It's not her oncologist. They are short one physician and have redistributed the patient load among the rest. He examines my sister's legs, reviews her file. "Why stop your chemo treatments, it can prolong your life?" he comments.

"It makes me very sick and the doctors tell me it won't prolong my life. If this is quality of life, I don't want it."

He's confused with the latest test results. He leaves us and returns moments later with Carmen's oncologist so he may continue the examination. Carmen is happy to see him. She prefers it this way.

Dr. Jones completes a requisition for more tests and refers my sister to a neurologist. They discuss her chemo treatments. He explains the importance of taking them as recommended. "Today's a short one." She reluctantly agrees to continue her chemo.

Sitting in her reclining chair, Carmen carries on a conversation with the nurse. Her questioning reveals the nurse is not starting with the right drip bag. Carmen tells her they begin with the other solution and then they administer the chemo. The nurse disagrees. Carmen is persistent. The nurse asks a colleague. Not satisfied with her colleague's reply, she interrupts the pharmacist. "Yes" he says "You always start with the saline solution. Chemo is second followed by antinausea medicine."

Carmen is attentive to her medication. She knows what she is taking.

★ ★ ★

Roger is meeting with the board of the cooperative on a regular basis. They have major issues to deal with and most are too complex for members to understand. He works with the board for months, guiding and coaching them through the process. He needs to be patient, they are inexperienced and lack the necessary competencies. The many meetings, the long hours become fruitful. They see the progress.

There comes a time when the board needs to discuss the upcoming trial. The lawsuit against Carmen was initiated by the previous board and is still pending. They are incurring legal fees as a result. Roger is ready to provide them with the evidence, Carmen's defense, so they can make an informed decision having all facts before them.

I phone my sister; I want to know if she's still comfortable with this. If the board decides to continue with the lawsuit, their lawyer will have Carmen's defense in hand. Any lawyer's dream.

Although my sister appears stronger, psychologically she's not. I barely ask the question and she breaks down in tears. "I can't make any decisions. It's too hard," and she continues to cry.

We need to keep it simple. "OK sis, Roger will look after everything. We will deal with this as if it is our own situation. We won't discuss it with you until it's done." What bothers Carmen the most is her reputation.

Roger provides the board with the evidence. He hopes his efforts will pay off and the board will see the injustice. Included in the documentation are the various reports that note the exceptional contribution Carmen made during her tenure and in the different leadership roles she played.

July 23, 2012

Carmen can't be any happier. She sees a picture of Martin and Anne on Facebook. Anne thinks she found her match.

Carmen is so excited. Jokingly I tell her, "Stop questioning them. You are too much into their lives. Let them breathe." I add, "You are 59 years old, mind your own business." She laughs.

Later that afternoon, George finds Carmen on her couch sobbing, "If you only knew how much I'm suffering." To hear her speak those words just tears him apart. He feels helpless.

★ ★ ★

Carmen's birthday is approaching. She wants a pool party at my place. We arrange it for the weekend so Denise and some of her children can attend. Joanne sings to the tune of Sister Sledge ... *We are family* ... Carmen enjoys the gathering. She's calm and relaxed. She is proud of her children; Lisa is happily married to James and is expecting. Carmen talks to Lisa's stomach, "Hello Lucas. This is your grandmother." She looks up, "I know he can hear me."

Martin and Anne are in love, they look happy. Carmen whispers, "I've never seen Martin so affectionate." She turns around and shouts, "Are you two going to wait until I die to get married?" We all laugh.

August 1st is the official day – she is 60 years old. We have a third birthday celebration for Carmen. We meet at her place for a BBQ with friends and neighbours. It will be her last.

"My neighbour's daughter is having a garage sale. I bought a crib, a high chair, a small bath and a few other baby items. It will be delivered tomorrow." Carmen tells me.

"For Lisa?"

"No. I want a baby room for when she visits."

George and I spend the next day cleaning and reorganizing Carmen's spare bedroom. She lies on the bed directing. We add a few stuffed animals to the crib. The room looks great.

Lisa phones me. She is uncomfortable with the possibility of her mother in the delivery room. "It's my first baby. I don't know what to expect and I'll be worried about my mom. She tires easily. She's often in pain. I don't know how long it will take for the baby." She continues, "I know this means so much to her. I want her to be there with us but she's very sick. I'm stressed."

I phone Carmen and share with her that I do not want to attend the birth. She is not pleased "Why?" she asks abruptly.

"I just don't think it's my place."

She snaps, "Then, I'll go by myself if I have to."

I reason with her, "You can't do that. You can't go by yourself. What if you need help? She could be in labour for hours, no one knows. What if she has complications? You don't want to be there for that. You can't sit that long. Why don't you go once the baby is born? Besides, it's really between the couple." I add jokingly, "You're 60 years old. You should mind your own business." My sister agrees it's probably best to wait until baby Lucas is born. "I want to be first at the door." It's not a request. It's a command.

I text Lisa, "You owe me another one, kiddo."

★ ★ ★

Although Carmen would often begin her day in tears, she was strong enough to allow herself time to mourn and then pull herself together. "I give myself five minutes a day," she would repeat. Most days it would be more.

It's early morning, Denise finds Carmen sitting on the couch wrapped in her favorite housecoat. She's holding a Kleenex in one hand and a few soiled ones in the other. Tears are rolling down her cheeks as she speaks. Her voice is breaking "Where am I going Denise? Where am I going?"

TRAVEL PLANS

It's August 2012. It's been 11 months. I made myself readily available to Carmen at all times. My cell phone accompanies me everywhere. Carmen's link to the outside world is her telephone. It is her social tool. It had been throughout her entire life. It is even more so this past year.

"I can't take her calling me five-ten-fifteen times a day. I can't take it anymore. It's the same conversations over and over again. I can't bear to hear my phone ring." I regret sharing my frustrations with Joanne and Roger. How could such words escape my lips? Obviously not one of my better moments. I'm not in a good place this week. Hopefully, not to be repeated. I definitely need my yoga practice and meditation. I need "normal" again. My assessment? Maybe I find the load too heavy … maybe others could do more … maybe I don't want to say goodbye … maybe I'm scared … maybe I don't want to live this. MAYBE! MAYBE! MAYBE! I learn to mince my words. They say to journal but I can't. I remind myself that I am the one responsible for my happiness.

I don't speak of what I'm living with many people. I'm not unique. It seems people tend to mourn privately. We become closet grievers. It's not to be brave or stoic. You simply sense the discomfort in people. It's evident by their facial expressions or their absence. Words of encouragement are difficult to come by. You also want to discuss other topics. Your mind needs to focus on something other than cancer and death.

You don't want to be repetitive, which can easily occur, given that it is a prolonged process. No doubt it's more comfortable discussing the topic with someone with similar experiences. I've come to the conclusion that if you have never experienced the role of a caregiver for a patient with a terminal illness – you really do not understand. It's a subject many have no knowledge of. It's more than just preparing meals, cleaning their house, doing their errands and accompanying your loved one to medical appointments; it's also the psychological and emotional support, the stress, the loving and caring on a daily basis. It's being there. It's managing your mourning, not quite understanding your feelings and those around you, while caring for someone you love and watching them suffer. It's with you 24 hours a day, seven days a week.

Depending on your role and support, you can easily burn out. It does take its toll. I know I need to create balance in my life. I am retired, I am available at all times but I also don't have work to distract me. Who determines who does what and when? It may not be obvious. Everyone has to be comfortable with the support they provide. Who is to say to the other you could do more? There's also a difference in the loss of a parent, a sibling, a child and a friend and how close the relationship you hold with the dying.

I feel somewhat restricted, although self-imposed. I feel I cannot share my frustrations with Carmen. I'm afraid if I do she will be offended and hurt, and may withdraw. Concerned it will make matters worse, I try to suppress my emotions. Given what she is living through – is it selfish of me? I need to get away. I too need to leave Cancerland.

Roger and I depart for Belgium and France for a three-week holiday in celebration of Roger's 60th birthday. No need to say it, I know my sister is not pleased with me leaving. During our absence, I communicate with Carmen by email. News is good – she had a great weekend with Denise, Sam and George. Her first grandson arrived one week early. My mother and her husband, Tim, were there hours after Lisa had given birth. Carmen bought an electric scooter. She had great news from her oncologist; her lymph nodes had decreased by 30%. All looked good during my absence, all, except they wanted her to start chemo again. She feels somewhat pressured by the medical staff.

★ ★ ★

Living in a different city, Mom is not able to see Carmen as often as the rest of us. She finds comfort hearing her voice. They speak daily. The conversations are brief. She can sense how her daughter is doing. When she worries about her, she phones the others to get the facts.

My mother is an emotional but strong woman. She lost most of her siblings to cancer or a heart condition, all in their early 60s. My dad died of cancer after 51 years of marriage. Her second husband is a cancer survivor. Mom was by Tim's side when he suffered from colon cancer and chemotherapy. "You never get used to it. But when it's your child, it's different. They are part of you regardless of their age. You don't expect to outlive your children."

Carmen does not want Mom to stay and care for her while we're away. "She's 80 years old; I have others to care for me."

August 22, 2012

The board made their decision in the absence of Roger. Based on the evidence, they withdraw the lawsuit, reimburse my sister for her legal fees and hand her an apology letter with a copy to each member of the cooperative. She is finally vindicated and her reputation restored. It is anticlimactic. I can't say my sister is happy. The decision comes in too late.

> **August 23, 2012**
> Carmen writes, "miss you my bosom".
>
> **August 24, 2012**
> Hey sis. We have a five-hour wait in Montreal. I forgot to tell you I have a crooked baby finger. I think it may be arthritis. Your hermana[10] Nicole. Luv u.
>
> **August 26, 2012**
> OK, we finally got to Brussels. We did not do much today because of jetlag. Lots of tourists. Leaving tomorrow for Brugges – a medieval town. We really enjoyed first class. How are we to sit in sardine class to come back home! Weather is about 17C & cloudy, which I don't mind.
>
> Hope you are having a good weekend with your other sister. Love you hermana. Nicole

---

[10] Spanish for sister

August 26, 2012
Had a nice weekend with Denise, we went to the casino Saturday. She is as much a black cloud as you are. She's in the black book for casino. We went to the Canadian Museum of Civilization and went to see the polar bears at IMAX. The Maya theme was not that interesting. They lent me a scooter while I was there – holy shit man I've got to get one of those. George did not have to pay because he was my escort, and we were all seniors so we got a reduction. George and Sam went biking Saturday from 9 A.M. to 8 P.M. and they left today at 4:30 P.M. George went shopping with Sam and bought a Lance Armstrong suit (skin tight pants; they lift the testicles) for his biking. Anyway, it did give him a nice weekend to do something different than to hear me nag. You could see how happy he was in his face. He might go in September. Sam is doing 50k for the firefighters so I will try to push him to go. I really feel better this week since I am not taking the chemo shit any more. Hope you are enjoying your trip. Denise said Hi. Write back sis, miss you. Oh, and tell Roger he is the only one for the casino. Carmen

August 27, 2012
There is a casino here in Brussels but Roger won't go because I'm here. And he says, "What were you thinking, going with a black cloud?" Hope you have money left for when we get back. He's getting worried.

Glad to hear you are feeling better and that you had a good weekend. Good too George went biking. It's great exercise; do encourage him to do the 50K with Sam.

Off to get our rental car. Will email you once in Brugges. Talk soon hermana favorita, Nicole XO

Forgot to ask if Mom has shingles or not.

August 27, 2012
She did not see the doctor. She told Denise she was coming

down the long weekend for a week. Have to call and get the story straight. Jennifer called her, she really wants to come down to visit me. I really don't see the point of her driving down and maybe seeing me for two hours. I don't want visitors who will sit on my couch for hours. I'm too sick. Tell Roger - better hurry back. I need money. I think I will buy a couch with my winnings. youpeeeeeeeeeeeee.

Miss you, love you *Por qué me dejaste*. Carmen

My reply
I am working on figuring out *dejaste*? I think me knows.

Jennifer may be there for hours. If you are too tired for visitors just tell her. Of course, I could simply mind my own business. After all, I am 52 and you are 60 (old enough to make your own decision) talk soon. luv u, Nicole

August 28, 2012
Por qué me dejaste means why did you leave me?

Later that day
Hi Hermana. Well, I just bought six bags of beets. Will be making my jars this Thursday. I feel much better since I am not taking any chemo. The only thing is my legs hurt so bad, my heel. The hospital phoned and left me a message that I had missed two appointments, and they scheduled me for the 5th and changed the time and to call them. Boy, did I call back. I told her I left messages with my nurse, and I am not responsible if she does not transfer her messages; and as for chemo on the 5th, I have a meeting at 2:30 P.M. with my oncologist to follow up on my scan. I don't want chemo. I will discuss it with my doctor. She says you have already missed two appointments. I told her - listen carefully, chemo makes me ill and I want to speak to my oncologist before. I am sick three weeks out of four, would you take the treatments? She replies no, I understand. Then I say - stop booking appointments! Miss you sis, love you. Carmen

I send her a long email from France on details of our trip. I add that I light candles for her when I visit cathedrals.

August 31, 2012
Sis, remember the image of Jesus Dad used to have. I think Mom gave you his prayer card. Well, I found this huge frame of the same image in a cathedral in the town of Honfleur (where Champlain initially left to discover Canada). So here I lit a candle for you and one for Dad. I always liked that image.

How are you feeling? What's going on? Next time we travel we'll set up Skype so we can talk online … well, if it works with our laptop in the country. We have a six hour time difference so I am now going to bed. Talk soon. Love you & miss you. Your bosom hermana. Say hi to everyone. Nicole

Carmen responds
Hi sis,

Nothing new. I did 24 jars of pickled beets. It took me two days. All is well. Mom should be coming down around September 6. Lisa is still waiting. She thinks her baby will have a cone head if he does not come out soon. Tell my casino friend I miss him. Glad you are enjoying your trip. Talk to you soon.

Love you hermana. Carmen

September 4, 2012
Mom is still in Welland; they are bringing the gas line to her new house. Lisa went to see the doctor; her labour has not started yet at all. Little Lucas is in no hurry to come and meet us. Martin and Anne are still in love. Went to see the neurologist this morning; he said the pain in my legs could be from the cancer but there were anomalies in my legs. He said they could insert a needle in my back and take liquid out and have it analyzed, and I told him I really don't see the point in doing that since I will not have any operations and the pain is not that bad. I kind of miss you guys. I will be having lunch Thursday with my beautiful goddaughter

Samantha and her boyfriend. She has moved back home with Joanne. I always have company every day so can't say I'm all by myself. I was very tired Sunday, I would have slept 24 hours. I am also tired today, don't know why and for sure I will be tired tomorrow. I will be seeing my oncologist so I am a bit nervous about what he might say, and I have to tell him I am not taking any more chemo. I also got a prescription for an electric chair or scooter from the neurologist today. Well, I miss you and I really need to go to the casino with my best buddy who will be turning 60 soon. Say hi to him and tell him I miss him. Love you lots sis. Hurry back home and I think the next time you plan a trip, I should be included in the discussions.

Love you hermana. Oh, did not get my money yet, everybody is sleeping on the $#$# thing.

September 5, 2012
A scooter? That would be pretty cool. Are you getting one? Good luck today with Dr. Jones. Will be thinking of you. I think I got Roger's bug.

Her reply
Yeah, today is the day; very, very nervous. If you would have stayed home you would not have had the bug, so no sympathy from me. I miss you. The chair of the board called their lawyer and he claims my lawyer did not send anything so no cheque for me. Phoned my lawyer three times never returned my call. I will try again today to see if it's true. I will go shopping for a scooter, today maybe. Tomorrow I go to lunch with Samantha and her boyfriend.

September 5, 201
Carmen sends me a picture of her on a scooter and adds, "I have called every day, even left a message that I need to buy a wheelchair and it would be nice to get my money."

September 6, 2012
Hi Sis,

Good news, went to the doctor he told me my lymph nodes had shrunk 30%. Said it was sad I had decided to quit. I told him I was sick three out of four weeks and he had told me it could not prolong my life. He told me the chemo was to shrink the lymph nodes and to prevent the cancer from spreading elsewhere like my brain etc. ... He said nobody can say how long I have, the cancer can be sleeping, could be one year or even five years. He said I only had three treatments to do. It was my decision but if I would not have taken the first three treatments, the lymph nodes would have swollen more and spread and probably choked me. So I nearly barfed. I told him I would take the last three. Starting next week I am scheduled, so let's hope for the best. Will start doing my mmmmmmmmmmmmmmthing. Went shopping for a scooter; holy shit it's as expensive as a motorcycle; of course, I picked the nicest one. Will send the claim to my insurance to see if they will cover the cost of $5000. Hope you are having fun. Miss you guys. Carmen

My response
Hi sis,

That is good news. The treatments are making a difference. Although you are sick, your body seems to react well to the treatments. Three more to go; you are half way through.

I know you don't care about my bug but I think it's finally gone. I have moved away from the toilet to the living room. But my baby finger is still swollen – it may be arthritis.

We did not do anything yesterday because I was sick. Today we visit the castle and the Leonardo deVinci museum. Tomorrow we leave for vineyards and our next phase of the trip, Burgundy. You must be really happy with your oncologist. Talk soon sis. Luv you.

Her reply
Sorry, did you have a bug? Can't wait to see that finger, maybe it's your imagination.

September 9, 2012
Well, George left yesterday for St-Sauveur to do the 50k with Sam. Seemed quite excited so I hope they have a great day. Feel a bit depressed that I have to take those treatments. I don't really have to, but it might prevent it from spreading and the lymph nodes had shrunk. I just think about it and feel like throwing up. No activity on Lucas' part. I have a feeling it could be this week but he will probably make a liar out of me. Mom did not come down yet but maybe next week. Joanne really loved my beets. Thought she did not like it but whatever, will make another batch today so you can have at least six jars for the winter in case you hibernate. Tell Roger I miss him and I miss you. Love you hermana, come back home.

My reply
I get six jars? Really? I love your beets. I'm so excited! I'm sure it will make a difference to George to do the 50K. He should have a good time.

You only have two-three treatments left. Take the nausea pills you are supposed to, even if you don't feel sick. It will go by faster than you think. Besides, since you have been taking that type of chemo, you have stopped coughing. Both I and your friend Donna noticed, so something is going right.

We just got into the Burgundy area today. We have a nice apartment only we can't figure out how to change the language on the TV from German. I'm learning lots for my wine program. We have put on close to 3,000 kilometres. I think I have blisters on my bum so don't ask me to take you for a ride when I get back.

I too think Lucas will come out this week. Miss you too but I think you don't write that often. BTW, my baby finger is still swollen and crooked. Talk soon sis. XO from both of us (Roger will be ready).

Marie and her husband meet Carmen, George, Mom and Tim for brunch. She also has terminal lung cancer – stage IV. Her prognosis is three to four months. She has been crying ever since she received her diagnosis. She is a wonderful woman, a friend of Mom and Tim. Carmen and Marie spoke many times by phone. They were looking forward to meeting. They have much in common. They understand each other. Carmen is a great support to her.

The suffering and fighting requires constant effort. My sister is making her own travel plans.

IT'S TIME

September 11, 2012
Today is Roger's 60th birthday. From Burgundy, France I email Lisa.

> "If you are not busy giving birth today and have a few moments to spare … can I ask a favour? Can you phone … on my behalf? I would like to sign up for …"

This generation is so wired they do nothing without their cell. I'm guaranteed a reply. She responds immediately.

> "Actually I AM giving birth today. I asked my mom to call for you. My water broke at 5:30 this morning. We went to the hospital. I don't really have contractions so they sent us home. We go back at 5:30 tonight for induction if nothing is happening. Happy Birthday Roger."

I am mostly excited for my sister. I pray everything will go well.

> **To Nicole**
> Hi sis, my computer was down but it's back up, the power supply died. Sent Roger a birthday card, hope he gets it. Little Lucas is trying to come out today, let's hope it works. Lisa will leave at 4 P.M. for supper and then the hospital. I'm starting the chemo tomorrow, hope I'm OK to see him. I'll drag the body if I have to. Give a kiss to Roger for his birthday. Mom should be coming down at the end of the week, good timing – she will see little Lucas. Love you and miss you xxxooo. Carmen

To Carmen

I phoned you about 20 minutes ago – no answer; so I texted Martin – he's good to reply immediately. I am so excited for all of you. But it's taking him a long time! We know he is slow and hard-headed! (Good start) If you don't have access to your emails, text me with George's cell phone. I can't wait for you to confirm he's gorgeous. Martin seems pretty excited. I think Martin will love him as much as I love yours. See you soon sis.

With all the excitement, your treatments will become secondary. You will be too busy thinking about Lucas etc. Great Mom is coming down at the same time, she loves babies. I wait for news. Good luck tomorrow. Take care. Love you.

It was not so long ago we never thought this would happen ... Nicole

To Nicole

Well, it's seven o'clock and still no Lucas. Lisa is in her room at the hospital, the doctor will see her around 7:30 P.M.; of course, her cell does not work too well, the reception, you know. So I asked her, do they not have a phone in the room? She said yes but they have to pay, so I said I will pay the darn phone, just hook it up! Chemo is still there, shit, tomorrow noon. Hope I am OK to see Lucas. It takes forever when you go to the hospital. You walk in at noon for your chemo treatment and out at 5 or 6 P.M. Sent Roger a birthday card, hope he gets it, listen to the music it says, "Roger". If he doesn't get it, let me know and I will send it to you.

Once I know Lucas popped his head out to meet the parents, will send you an email.

Love, miss you. I think you are mean leaving me for such a long time. I thought you loved me. Carmen

To Carmen
It's 5:22 P.M. at this end. Has he arrived? You up? Nicole

To Nicole
I haven't slept yet. It's 4 A.M. really tired, can't sleep - fuc^%^ chemo and waiting for Lucas. Have not heard anything yet, maybe they didn't want to call. I will call them around 7:30 A.M. I am soooooooo tired.

Carmen dreads every single one of her chemo treatments. Toxic chemicals being administered intravenously into her body, accumulating with every dose. The side effects of the last chemo treatment barely decrease and another treatment commences. She fears the side effects. The appointment to the hospital is tiring in itself; it takes the day and all her energy. She regrets ever starting chemotherapy but she feels pressure. She fears suffering. If she abandons, is she giving up? Maybe the treatments will prolong her life.

To Carmen
Go for a nap on your couch. They will call you when he arrives. You are probably too excited about the baby. It usually took a few days for you to feel at your worst from the side effects of your treatments. Nicole

We exchange a few more emails while waiting for little Lucas to arrive.

Hey sis, Do you recall when we were trying to guess the date of birth … you, me and Lisa? And we thought the 12th was a good date. Funny huh. Nicole

… Martin and Anne are in LOVE and I luv you. Carmen

Baby Lucas arrives. My sister is in heaven … well not yet, but at least on cloud nine.

September 12, 2012
To Nicole – Well, Mr. Lucas was born at 7:29 A.M. Mother and father are doing well. Lucas has a lot of dark hair just like his godfather and he has Lisa's little dimple in the chin. They do not know how much he weighs yet. Will be visiting after my chemo.

Lisa had to push for two hours and they had to take the suction cup to pull him out. James said they were doing a lot of stitches down there, ouch! Will keep you posted. Mom is coming tomorrow. Love and miss you, Carmen

"Give him to me, give him to me," my sister shouts as she sprints into the maternity room.

It had to take all of Carmen's energy to make it from one hospital to another. They sent me a photo of her holding her grandson. The photo speaks for itself. My sister's face is glowing – she is so happy; she is so proud. It's a lovely picture.

> **To Nicole**
> He is gorgeous. I had this fatigue and I do look tired but I had to go today. I had to see him. Lisa looked very tired, they did not sleep and boy, she did feel the pain, thought she was dying. She had to push for two hours with big pain and has a lot of stitches, she's very sore. Carmen

Pictures continue coming in by cell and by email. In one of my congratulatory emails to Lisa and James, I include … "Imagine when you were born that's how much your mother loved you. How nice is that!"

> **To Carmen**
> Thank God our plans changed and we were not standing there! How are you feeling today? I got this lingering kind of cold. I hope it clears by the time I take my plane … Love you. Nicole

> **September 13, 2012**
> **To Nicole**
> Yeah, lucky we were not there. I would have been very upset to see that and I would probably have sent you to get the doctor (hihi), you know, since I'm handicapped. He is so beautiful. I really could put him in a duffle bag and bring him home with me…. Love you and miss you. Carmen
>
> p.s. went to bed at 1 A.M. and woke up at 5 A.M. - very nauseous, so took a gravol - it's not too bad now.

Lisa phoned me this morning, said she slept well. She woke up every three hours to feed Lucas. When she was talking to me he was waking up, you could hear the little cry in the background. She will be going home today. So if Mom arrives early I will go with her to the hospital. If she arrives late, well, I will go for an hour and we will visit Lisa Friday or Saturday. Carmen

September 15, 2012
To Carmen
…How are you feeling? News please.
Congratulations! Love you. Nicole

Carmen's reply
Did you get the picture of me and Mom with Lucas? Have been pretty busy with your mother. Haven't stopped since the chemo. I'm dragging my ass. Going to Lisa's this afternoon with Mom, Joanne, Tim and Pappi George, then going to Red Lobster for supper. Mom is leaving tomorrow probably. I will try to meet her friend Marie tomorrow after church. He is so gorgeous. I love him sooooooo much. I do miss my bosom but you don't write back.

September 17, 2012
I'm coming home sis! … love you. Nicole

I find little decline in Carmen's health once we're back home. In fact, she looks better than other times during her chemo treatments. I thought it was strange that she did not visit her little grandson more often. Perhaps it's due to Lisa's fatigue and her own. Mother and daughter have something more in common.

Carmen is thrilled with Lisa's unexpected visit; a surprise visit with her grandson. I wonder if all grandmothers are that proud.

"She's a good mother." She tells me, "I knew she would be."

A few days later Carmen, George and I were to meet at Lisa's to visit Lucas. I arrived 30 minutes early to surprise my sister and to hold the baby before she arrived. This way, she could have him all to herself during her visit. My sister saw it differently. She continuously asked George and me to take the baby. She wants us to love him. "We do love him," I say. But she wants us to love him more. She later shares with me her arms are weak. She cannot hold little Lucas even when the baby is resting on the breastfeeding cushion. Lucas is barely seven pounds.

The living room is comfortably warm. Carmen has chills. She feels a cold coming on. Minutes later, James arrives - he left work early. He removes his shoes and walks directly up the stairs to his bedroom. He is sick as a dog with an awful cold.

Prior to her cancer, if you mentioned the word "cold": Carmen would get one. Today, she is catching one. Her immune system is weak, leaving her body vulnerable to infection, a side effect of chemo.

Although it is suggested that one avoid crowds and public places while undergoing chemo treatments, Carmen went to the casino with her gambling partner Roger the day before. She could have gotten this bug anywhere.

★ ★ ★

It's September 24th, my father died this day 13 years ago. He was 73. His younger sister Juliette was with us that morning. We were all gathered in my dad's hospital room. Before leaving the hospital, Aunt Juliette asked that we phone her at 4 P.M. He died at that exact time – 4 P.M. September 24, 1999. I always said he called her directly.

The sisters get together to visit Dad's grave two years after his passing. We drive five-hours to the cemetery. At the gate entrance we find bright plastic flowers on top of the garbage can. We always teased Dad that we would plant tacky plastic flowers. Is it a coincidence these flowers were presented to us? They look new. We plant them. We laugh. We continue on to Sudbury for the night. The next morning we stop at the cemetery again en route home. As we drive off, we spot a bear cub in the adjacent field. We park the car and wait to see what he will do. We never saw the mother bear. We return to Ottawa. It was George who said, maybe it's your father – the flowers, Tinour.

On this anniversary Denise sends us an early morning email regarding Dad's passing. The rest of us had forgotten (temporarily I'm sure), even Carmen, which is unusual.

Carmen phones Denise. She wants her to come down on Wednesday. She continues to feel ill but wants a get-together at her place. She's disappointed to hear I'm going to Toronto that morning to play golf. She insists she wants Denise to meet Lucas for the first time. She wants her to bring her iPad to take pictures. Denise hesitates; she has such a busy week. She rearranges her schedule.

The previous Friday, Carmen cancelled her weekend with Denise and Sam. She was tired, weak and felt like she was catching a cold – all common side effects of chemo. Side effects she's had multiple times. The forecast was heavy rain for the weekend. I encouraged her to rest.

Carmen returns home after a visit to her family physician. Her cold has turned to pneumonia. Lisa calls everyone. The get-together is cancelled. She needs to rest. Everyone is notified except for Denise. Carmen waits until her older sister is in town before dialing her cell number.

"Stop in at Jean Coutu Pharmacy to get a face mask. I don't have the energy to search for my box in the apartment. I don't know where they are. I don't want to give you a cold."

Denise walks into the apartment wearing a mask. They don't kiss because Carmen has pneumonia. She sits next to her on the couch. The mask continuously fogs up her glasses. Denise eventually removes it. They share peanuts from the same bag. Carmen says "I didn't wash my hands."

"It's OK sis. I don't care if I get a cold. Are you hungry? Do you want me to make you a soup?"

"No, Martin will bring me some Chinese macaroni later in the afternoon." Carmen kept trying to find a comfortable position on her couch. She asks, "Is it possible to see dead people before you die?"

"Yes. Aunt Lora saw dead people. Do you see people? Who did you see?"

"Lots ... a lot of people. I don't know them all."

"Who did you see that you know?"

"Ron."

"Ron who?"

"My children's biological father."

"What did he say?"

"Nothing ... he sat next to me and softly rubbed my back and smiled at me." As she prepares to lie on her side she adds, "He looked better. He was handsome as I knew him when we were younger." She continues, "Do you want to ride my scooter?"

The television is on, Carmen sleeps for a while. Denise is still reflecting on Carmen's vision.

How strange. She eventually returns to her book.

Later that afternoon Denise warms a bowl of Tim Hortons tomato soup for Carmen. The coffee table is packed. She pushes aside the papers, Kleenex, inhalers, medications, finger oximeter, and candies to make room for the bowl. She doubts Carmen will eat it.

Carmen is extremely tired. She tells Denise, "If I go to bed early I will leave the lights and the television on. Simply turn everything off when you return from Anne's."

Before leaving, Denise rubs Carmen's back and chest with Vicks. She feels her ribs with every stroke. Denise leaves around 5 P.M. with Martin. Anne's apartment is a short drive away. Lisa joins them for dinner. Denise spends time filming Lucas.

George phones Carmen twice during the evening. There is no answer, she is in bed. He thinks she needs the rest. Denise will be there shortly.

Martin drives Denise back to the apartment. En route, she tells him about Carmen's vision. He returns to Anne's apartment, looking for Lisa. He finds her in the bedroom changing the baby's diaper. He quickly tells her about his conversation with Denise. Lisa interrupts him, "You are going to make me cry. Tell me no more. This is creepy."

The lights are on in the apartment. Carmen is in her bedroom. Denise assumes she is sleeping.

Denise phones me on my cell, we talk for a while. She finds Carmen has changed. I don't recall if she told me of the vision that night.

As soon as we hang up Denise hears a noise coming from the bedroom. She walks over and enters the room. Carmen wants water. She already has three glasses on her dresser. Her mouth feels dry and coated. She has an awful headache. Carmen is lying in bed naked. She's warm and perspiring; the hair on the back of her head is wet and curly. She wants two Ativan. "I need to sleep. I'm so tired," she says.

The room is dark. Denise can't see her clearly but finds she looks strange. She phones George from the kitchen. There's no answer. She returns with the water and turns on the light in the hallway. Carmen does not look good.

Carmen asks, "Did George call? Do we call George? Maybe he called." George is her security blanket, ours as well.

Denise offers to phone him.

"He's probably sleeping," Carmen says.

"No, it's too early." Denise tries the cordless phones resting on the bed. All three are dead. She calls George with her cell. He is on his way.

Denise lies down next to Carmen. She takes her iPad and begins going through the pictures she took of Lucas. "He is beautiful, isn't he?" Carmen says proudly.

"Yes, he's a beautiful baby."

Carmen is holding her head. Her headache prevents her from continuing to browse at photos. George walks in. He finds Carmen is not looking well. He turns on the bedroom light. He suggests they take her to the hospital.

She doesn't want to hear anything about it. "I'm too tired. If I'm not feeling better tomorrow morning, we can go then."

They try to convince her it would be better. Denise says, "Carmen, you are suffering. You have an awful headache. They could give you something to kill the pain. You will be in good hands. You don't look very good."

She finally agrees. George goes into the kitchen to dial 911. The clock on the microwave reads 9:36 P.M. He returns to dress Carmen.

In the meantime, Denise is searching for the diapers. Carmen is sitting on the edge of the bed asking impatiently and repeatedly for one. Several soiled diapers are left on the floor. Probably ones she tossed aside during the night.

George knows where to go. He pulls out a diaper, grabs Carmen and lifts her. He slides the diaper under her behind. She doesn't even have to get up. They have the routine down pat.

Denise is anxious. She is pacing the hallway waiting for the ambulance, and occasionally stands in the bedroom doorway watching the drama unfold.

George pulls a bra from Carmen's dresser. "No," she says as she waves her arm in disgust, "I don't want to wear a bra." He puts it back in the drawer and reaches for her pajama top. Like a child, she lifts both arms straight up in the air and he slides it on. He slips on her pajama bottom, both legs at once. He lifts her again to finish the job. He proceeds with the socks.

Denise continues her pacing. She is now in the living room. Carmen arrives, sitting in her wheelchair, George pushing from behind. They can see the ambulance through the window. The emergency lights are on but not the sirens. George returns to the bedroom to collect a few things. He tells Denise she is standing at the wrong door; they will be coming in from the other entrance.

The two paramedics enter with a stretcher. The one with the Iroquois haircut has a few tattoos and body piercings in the face. He approaches Carmen, "So, what's wrong my little Madame?"

She snaps, "Well! I have cancer. I'm at stage IV. I have a headache. I'm nauseous. I don't feel well!"

He maintains the conversation by asking her what medication she took while they move her unto the stretcher. She lists them all. They adjust the backrest and lock it at a 65° angle. They begin checking her vital signs. He informs her she has to bring all her medication.

George returns from the bedroom with Carmen's purse and grabs the zip lock bag containing her meds. The medic instructs George to turn off the oxygen concentrator as he places the oxygen face mask on Carmen.

"We usually don't," he says.

The medic tells him it's best. The apartment instantly becomes quiet.

Denise is texting me. "Who are you texting? I told you not to call the kids. They don't need to worry." Carmen's hearing is particularly vibrant.

The medics roll the stretcher out of the apartment and then lift it up the three stairs toward the ambulance. Carmen is waiting for them to open the doors. George and Denise follow. The apartment door locks behind them. The neighbours are standing in their windows observing. They don't know this is the last time they will see her alive.

A family member is not allowed in the ambulance, unlike in the movies. Denise and George trail behind in Denise's van. They drive to the Gatineau Hospital and park at the pharmacy across the street. It will be faster than waiting to park at the hospital, going through the gates for a ticket and then finding a parking spot.

This hospital houses the regional Cancer Centre as their major specialty. The same one Carmen attends for her consultations and treatments. Denise and George enter through the Emergency Department. Carmen is on the stretcher. She is very agitated. The medics are in the process of transferring her to the nurse. They call out the vital signs. She is looked after quickly and moved from the stretcher to a bed in the Emergency Department. Carmen lists all the medication she's taken today; she also adds the type of chemo treatments she's on. The nurse records the information. My sister is very lucid.

Carmen is restless. She turns from side to side, she's not comfortable. Her oxygen nasal tube keeps slipping. George tries to adjust it. The hospital quarters are tight. The beds are lined up closely together, separated by a curtain with little room to stand next to Carmen. There is no room for visitors, nowhere to sit.

The nurse invites them to the waiting room. "There is nothing we can do until the physician arrives. Only he can decide the tests required." In the meantime, the nurse increases Carmen's oxygen level. George puts a wet face cloth on Carmen's forehead. Denise and George take turns checking in and staying with Carmen. They were there for hours. Carmen's fatigue is evident. They give her a sedative to calm her. They eventually send her for an X-ray.

George and Denise are in the waiting room. The physician enters, calling for the Miller family. He tells them, "She is not leaving here." They interpret this as she is staying overnight, maybe a few days. He proceeds, "Have you had any discussions regarding resuscitation? In her condition, we can easily break a few ribs. Patients suffer much more afterwards."

George and Denise look at each other. Both are surprised at the question and don't know what to reply. They are not sure why he is asking. He doesn't say.

George mentions he wants to speak with Roger. "He was the CEO of a hospital in Ottawa …" Denise realizes he is lost. What's Roger got to do with this? She tells the physician she is not aware of Carmen's decision, but maybe she discussed it with me, or her son.

It's a quarter to one in the morning. Denise can't reach me. She decides to contact Martin regardless of Carmen's wishes.

"Martin, your mother is in the hospital. It's not going well …" She goes on but he's half asleep. He's not sure what to think. "OK. Should I come down? Maybe call me when you have more news …"

Denise continues, "They have questions we can't answer. Decisions need to be taken. I can call you back in 15 minutes. They are currently administering medication by intravenous."

Denise and George are not aware of the medication being administered in the hospital. They are told it will take two to three hours to empty the bag of serum. The nurse suggests they take the time to rest. "It could be a while. Once the bag is empty, the physician will determine what additional tests are required."

Martin goes to the washroom after the call. Anne waits for him in the living room. "We can't really go back to bed. We might as well go to the hospital." They pick up Tim Hortons coffee for the group and arrive near 1:30 A.M.

The four of them wait. They debrief on their earlier conversation with the physician.

Carmen is less agitated. The nurse again wants the family to return to the waiting room. Carmen is lying on her left side in a fetal position with her right arm extended over the railing and covering her face. Denise kisses her arm. "I love you sis. We will come back later. Martin and Anne will stay with you."

Carmen responds with a, "hmmmm". Martin and Anne stay at the hospital. Denise and George leave around 3 A.M. They will rest and return later.

Martin looks at his mother. He does not speak to her. He does not wake her. He returns to the waiting room. He later shares with a nurse his mother's wishes. As with Denise and George, he is oblivious to what's happening.

The hospital staff is not sharing much information. Either they are not proactive or simply clueless about a patient's physical condition when approaching end-of-life. Could the latter be possible? I doubt it, given the physician's earlier question.

The nurse indicates the test results should be available around 4:45 A.M. when the physician does his rounds. Martin is told he is the only physician in the hospital. It's common knowledge that physicians sleep during the graveyard shift. Maybe that's where he was off to.

George returns to his apartment and Denise to Carmen's. It is dead quiet. The oxygen concentrator is off. The apartment is cold. Denise rests on the bed fully clothed. She is not sleeping well.

At 4:45 A.M. a voice over the intercom resonates throughout the emergency waiting room, "THE MILLER FAMILY TO TRIAGE DOOR #2, PLEASE."

As Martin and Anne make their way through door #2, a nurse is standing, waiting for them. They follow her through a different exit and a corridor until they reach two glass doors – **TRAUMA ROOM** – written in large, black bold letters.

A chill penetrates Martin's body as he reads the sign, every letter a focal point. He senses what is coming. The nurse's hand covers a red button and the automatic doors slide open. The room is crowded. On the left side the physician is standing, leaning against a desk, waiting to ask the question. On the right side of the room, Carmen is lying in a bed, barely visible with her oxygen mask, tubes, flashing monitors and equipment. She is surrounded by seven or eight people waiting for orders to resuscitate. One individual is continuously pumping a small black rubber oxygen bag connected to Carmen's face mask.

The physician directs his question to Martin, "Do we let her go? Or do we resuscitate your mother?"

Martin looks at his mother. Tears begin rolling down his cheeks. In a low, soft voice he responds, "Let her go." He tilts his head, he looks at nothing.

The physician waves his hand with his index finger pointing towards the door, a motion directing the team to leave. He shares with Martin that it is the most humane decision he could take. He follows his team out of the room. A nurse stays behind. She begins disconnecting the equipment, the tubes and connecting wires. She removes Carmen's oxygen mask and turns off the monitors and the oxygen. The room falls silent.

Carmen is left to breathe on her own. Anne and Martin are next to her. Anne directs her question to the nurse, "How much time do we have? Can we call people?"

"Minutes … actually, it could be seconds," as she makes her way to the desk.

While Martin is holding his mother's hand, Anne strokes her hair. She then walks to the nurse's desk located within the trauma room and makes a few phone calls on behalf of Martin.

"Denise, it's Anne. It's not looking good. If you want to see Carmen you have to come now. I tried to reach George but there is no answer." Denise keeps asking questions, had they spoken to the physician? Anne wants to leave things vague. She does not want to cause a panic. She recalls when she was driving at 160 km/hr trying to get to a hospital for a sick relative a long time ago.

George finally answers. "Get dressed," Denise orders, "it's not going well for Carmen." The two of them drive back to the hospital. A *déjà vu* all over again – this one with a twist.

Carmen is still alive. Martin continues to hold her hand; he gently touches her face, her hair. "We could not ask for a better mother … I love you, Mom."

He nods to Anne's next question, "Should I contact Lisa?"

She's hoping James will answer.

The phone rings. Lisa knows a call at that hour must be about her mother. She jumps out of bed to answer. Anne wants to speak to James, she asks twice to be transferred. Lisa refuses, "No. Tell me what's going on. Is it my mom?"

"Yes, we are at the hospital," Anne is uncomfortable.

"Is she dead? Is she OK?" Ever since Carmen was diagnosed, Lisa has been expecting this call.

"I don't know. Humm … they say it's over. It's not going well."

Lisa wants to vomit. She hangs up confused. She's not quite sure if her mother is dead or not.

Earlier that morning, around 1 A.M., Lisa is breastfeeding and reflecting on her earlier conversation with Martin. How long after you see dead people do you die? The light in the baby's room flickers a few times – it never does. She thinks maybe it's Ron, her father. It must mean something when dying people see dead people.

Confused Lisa runs to the guest bedroom to wake up James. They have been sleeping apart for a week because of his cold.

"We have to go to the hospital."

"OK. What's going on?"

"I don't know. I feel like I don't know what's going on. Anne said it's over. I don't know if my mom is dead."

Lucas is two weeks old. Lisa has not been sleeping much. No one wanted to stress her during her pregnancy and even less so with a newborn.

Anne returns to Carmen's bedside. She missed her last breath by seconds.

"She's gone. Her last breath was smooth, hardly noticeable. The next one never came. She simply stopped breathing." Martin continues to cry.

The two are standing next to Carmen, weeping in each other's arms. The nurse remains at her desk working on her files.

In all, they barely had ten minutes with Carmen. Everything afterwards became a blur. Anne and Martin take turns stepping out of the room to greet people as they arrive. They never felt Carmen's spirit that day.

Lisa wakes Lucas to feed him before leaving. The phone rings again. Martin is crying.

Lisa is confused, "What's going on?"

"Mom is dead."

"What the hell happened? What's going on?"

Martin explains. Lisa wishes they had phoned earlier. She is so tired – it's hard having a baby – the lack of sleep, the emotions, and her hormones were out of whack.

She is concerned about seeing her mother's dead body. She remembers how hard it was seeing my dad, her grandfather, in his coffin. I recall her pain that day. That's when I told Carmen, "We have been so busy with ourselves, we have forgotten to prepare the kids."

James tries to comfort Lisa. He's been through this himself two years ago when his father died of a heart attack. He explains seeing his father's body helped bring closure.

By the time they arrive, everyone is surrounding Carmen. Lisa manages to greet and hug everyone without looking at her mother. Only when she reaches George can she clearly see her mother's face. She then walks to the other side of the curtain. Although she can feel her mother's presence, her spirit, she cannot bear to look at her lifeless body. For a long time she holds that image in her mind.

Such images disappear with time. We no longer see our loved ones as the sick people they were. We eventually remember them when they were healthy. I always jolt when I see a photo of my dad or Carmen when they were very ill. I would rather not see such pictures, it saddens me and I feel for them. I can meticulously describe their appearance during that time but my mind seems to retain a healthy picture of them.

We imagine Carmen surrounded by family for her passing. We loved her and wanted to be by her side for these precious moments.

It is unfortunate the physician in charge was not clear in his communication. It is unfortunate he did not understand the value and role of family at end-of-life. The same for the emergency personnel, it is unfortunate no one took that extra step. Dr. Elisabeth Kübler-Ross would be disappointed.

Ironically, the physicians constantly reminded my sister she was dying of cancer from the very beginning. We heard it on many occasions during the last year. Strange when the time arrives, the physician's lips never pronounce the words death or dying. The family is in a different state of mind, oblivious to what is happening, relying on the medical staff. They need to hear the words clearly and directly. No one knows exactly when one will depart, but you do know it's approaching.

Had the family known it was Carmen's last day, or any indication it was coming, we would have been by her side for her last six hours instead of sitting in the emergency ward waiting, or elsewhere. You wonder, if the physician never had to ask the question about resuscitation, when would the family have been notified, after her passing? We are thankful she was not alone when she left this world, if merely for a few minutes.

When my father was dying, the hospital personnel had transferred him in a private room with space and chairs for the family to accompany him as he left us for the next world. We spent his last 24 hours together. We are grateful for such caring and compassionate health care providers. They should be proud.

It's not only coming to and witnessing your loved one's last breath as much as the hours following their passing that are precious. You feel the spirit, the life, the energy as it leaves the body. An intense sensation of peace and love fill the room. These are precious moments shared with the dying, with the family and with friends. Do not rob them of this opportunity.

Things were going well. Before her pneumonia, Carmen looked better than she did most times during her chemo treatments.

It never crossed my mind to ask my sister if she was transitioning that week. I never thought of asking if she felt she was approaching death. I didn't think she was at that stage. I was expecting her to die once she lost her full autonomy, once she was bedridden, similarly to the way my dad passed away.

I wonder if she actually knew – she never said.

It's been one year practically to the day of her diagnosis and in accordance with the physician's prognosis. My father's prognosis was eight months and he survived 11. Marie was given three to four months and she lived five. All three had terminal lung cancer, stage IV.

I wonder if Carmen sensed I abandoned her. My going to Toronto - was it really necessary? Maybe she sensed my frustrations and my need for travel. I know she thought George deserved more in life than this. She was concerned about him. She leaves in peace knowing her children are well taken care of. Both have a new love in their life.

Something I learned through my readings (post my sister's passing) is when a terminally ill patient asks you to come, you do so; otherwise it may be too late. I like to think they know their time. I pretend they have some control.

How many times do I hear myself saying, "They choose when they leave." How many times do you hear of people dying from chemo or complications, but not the cancer?

Carmen left. Not according to my plan – but she left. She did so leaving us with a special gift. She helped us grow. I miss her so.

I did not invite my sister to my wedding (my elopement). She did not invite me to her passing. I can hear Carmen's laughter as she reads these words.

My sister is ready … I wonder if she told Him … it's time.

SAYING GOODBYE

You are never ready. It comes fast and by surprise.

September 27, 2012

My father was buried 13 years ago on this day.

4:53 A.M.

As Roger and I leave Toronto and take the 401 East to Ottawa, I text Martin and Denise "We r on our way. Tell her I luv her."

4:54 A.M.

Martin responds, "OK, she loves you too."

The time of death was recorded as **4:55 A.M.** Did Martin ever read her my text? I know later she could not have replied. But did he tell her?

Denise phones me. She and George are en route to the hospital. "Carmen is very weak and won't be coming out of the hospital." My immediate thought – she is dying! I'm surprised no one else was contacted. But yet Carmen had such a hold on people when she wanted to. Again, they were given strict instructions not to tell anyone she was in the hospital.

I inform Denise I'll call everyone. She says, "Yes, to pray." I say, "To come down!"

Denise and George did not comprehend what the physician meant when he said, "She is not leaving here." They thought overnight or temporarily. After all, we have been through this before. It was not the first time Carmen went into the hospital for pneumonia.

I'm trying to reach Joanne but the line is busy. I proceed to wake Mom telling her it's not looking good. She will be coming down immediately. As I'm speaking with Karen another call comes in. I hang up to phone her later. It's Martin, sobbing; he tells me Carmen left us five minutes ago.

It's over. Just like that.

It all seems surreal. My sister is gone – my bosom friend. I feel frozen in time.

I'm sad I'm not there with her. I'm sad she is gone. I'm thankful Martin was by her side.

Martin had already called Joanne. I call David – he is also in shock. "I didn't know she was in the hospital. I didn't know this was happening." I reply, "We didn't either. She went in late last night. Her cold quickly turned to pneumonia. Her heart was too weak; it could no longer take it."

We are to contact him later once we know the funeral plans. He does not know if he will come today. He wants to see her. I reach Mom again, we cry together.

Regardless of whether Martin ever told her, I know Carmen read my text.

Joanne and Ken are on their way to the hospital. Anne had reached Lisa moments before. She was feeding Lucas and would leave shortly after. In subsequent discussions with Martin, I realize Lisa was not aware of her mother's passing. They simply told her Carmen was in the hospital and was very sick. I instructed Martin to phone her immediately. "She can't hear the news when she arrives at the hospital; she should know before – it needs to sink in. Sometimes, we can be too protective and make matters worse." He follows through.

I wait a few minutes and text Lisa, "I luv u. Give her a big hug." She replies, "Drive safe." I knew then she would find touching the dead odd and eerie. I hear later she could not look at Carmen in the hospital – this was not the mother she knew.

The sunrise is beautiful and dangerously blinding on the road. The highway is congested with transport trucks. Roger drives at a higher speed than his usual – over 135 km/hr. I cry most of the way. It seems to take forever. I text Martin, "Wait for me for funeral arrangements."

We finally make it to Ottawa in time for morning rush hour. The family is gathered at Carmen's apartment. We are just blocks away but we continue towards the hospital. I'm anxious to see her.

The hospital parking lot is practically full. We drive around to find a parking spot. The main entrance is relocated due to renovations. We make our way to the emergency ward.

We are told Carmen is in the morgue as we expected. The receptionist is kind and understanding; unfortunately, no one seems to be aware of the protocol. We wait over an hour in the emergency waiting room. The early sun is bright and shines through the glass wall – a new addition to the room.

A few families are waiting. They have their own crises to deal with. I get the occasional stare; it's evident I have been crying for hours. I'm one of those fortunate ones who looks bruised after a good cry. When you hurt, your looks are secondary.

The receptionist informs us throughout the hour that they are trying to find a manager to accompany us. She leaves for her morning break. Her replacement is not as compassionate. Roger's impatience is escalating. We are tired.

I approach the reception desk one last time. "And?" I say, "It's been over an hour. We are still waiting."

"It won't be long."

"I want to see my sister. What's the problem? What's so complicated?"

"Just another five minutes, Madame."

"We've been told 'five minutes' many times this past hour. I want to see her now. You realize I have many things to do. I don't need a manager to see her. Simply ask the security guard to unlock the door. I'm good with that."

He leaves his station and returns to eventually escort us to a small private waiting room. "Someone will be with you in a few minutes," and he leaves.

The room is cold in temperature and decor. I sit on a small black leatherette couch, Roger on the chair. I sense we are getting closer. It should not be long. We wait. After another 15 minutes, I make my way to the reception desk; he is not at his station. A security guard and manager are standing at the end of the corridor discussing – they realize I'm the one waiting; they tell me they are ready. I return with Roger.

Introductions are not required. We are escorted by the manager up a flight of stairs and then to the elevator. People are looking at me. I don't need a mirror. I know my eyes are swollen; my nose and face are red. My hair is probably a mess. Again, my looks are secondary. I don't pay attention. I don't care. We don't speak. We follow.

We arrive at a set of double doors. There is no indication this is the morgue. A sign "Restricted To Personnel Only" is posted on each door. We are asked to wait while they prepare my sister. It takes a few more minutes.

The ward is busy; people come and go. On several occasions, we take a step back to create space for the flow of traffic. Next to us, a husband repeatedly kisses his wife before the nurse wheels her off to the operating room. The floor is dirty. It could use a sweep.

The manager returns. The security guard unlocks the door. As we walk in, another guard pulls a yellow curtain creating a small private room and blocking the rest of the morgue from view.

On our right, Carmen is lying on a table. I hear myself saying, "Ahh, she is beautiful." Roger and I approach her body. I gently touch her face. I stroke her hair. Her body is cold. It is resting on the table as if in a coffin. A white sheet covers her body up to her shoulders. Only her face and neck are exposed. I feel the sheet to discover her hands are placed on her abdomen one on top of the other.

The guard is standing behind me; the manager on the other side of the curtain out of view; Roger on my right side. I begin to cry and so does Roger. From the corner of my eye, I see Roger turn towards the guard. I know a box of Kleenex is coming my way. I take a few. Roger does as well and deposits the box on my sister's stomach.

I kiss her forehead, I touch her arms, I remove my glasses before kissing her cheek, and I hug her. I talk to her silently – "I'm sorry sis, I'm so sorry I wasn't here for you. I love you."

I don't feel her spirit in the room.

I meticulously examine my sister. Her body is resting on bags of ice. A few bags are scattered over her body around her arms, all hidden from view under the white sheet. I could have stayed with her all day. She is so beautiful, she's at peace.

Her hair is straight again, salt and pepper. Her face is no longer swollen. Her skin has a grayish tint. Strangely enough, it appears somewhat natural. I recall Dad's was a glowing yellow. Her eyes are closed. Her upper and lower eyelids, the outer edges of her eyes are much darker, similar to people from the Middle East. Glue residue is visible between her lips. She has facial hair on her mole located just above her lip. I must tell Lisa. Carmen had ordered her daughter to remove any facial hair if ever she was in a nursing home and couldn't do it herself or if she was in a casket. She won't have to do it after all.

I gently stroke my sister's hair, kiss her one last time and proceed to leave the room, neglecting to give Roger his space. I hold off – he too has lost a friend.

The manager escorts us to the main entrance. We thank him and shake hands. It takes us over 15 minutes to exit the parking lot. It's bumper-to-bumper traffic. As usual, there's only the one attendant at the gate. As Roger pays the parking fee, they exchange words.

"Are senior management aware of the unacceptable delays and inefficiencies in the hospital parking system?" inquires Roger.

"Yes," the attendant replies.

"Good thing!"

We drive to Carmen's to spend the day with family, comforting each other. We hug everyone when we arrive. I walk into the room; Roger is behind me. Denise is first, then Joanne, followed by Anne, Martin and Ken. As I turn to my left to continue, George walks towards me. I open my arms to greet him and I hear Ken saying, "Here we go again; we are all going to start crying." George and I are about the same height, I can easily hold on to him. I don't let go.

"George, she was so beautiful. I caressed her. I kissed her. She is in peace."

I feel his cries, "I did as well, I caressed her and I kissed her. I did not stop."

We hold on tight as we sob in each other's arms. I find a closer bond with him, more than ever. I know he lost his greatest love.

Left sitting on the couch is Lisa, and then James, who is holding little Lucas in his arms. He is so tiny. As I approach Lisa, she gets up, "I'm glad you are here." We rock each other as we hug. I proceed to kiss James and Lucas.

I miss David. I wish he was with us. It must be more difficult for him to be without his siblings. My mother arrives a few hours later. She chooses not to visit the morgue. She prefers remembering Carmen as she saw her last, two weeks ago when Lucas was born.

I phone David. He is trying to close a real estate deal. I tell him we have 12 hours from the time of death to access the morgue. Given he has at least a five-hour drive, he would have to leave Kitchener shortly. He has until

5 P.M. today if he wants to see her. I describe the process. He calls a few hours later; he won't be coming up until the funeral.

★ ★ ★

When Denise and George arrived at the hospital that morning, they did what one does when you hear, "It's best if you come now … it does not look good." You drive in a haste and you race from the parking lot through the corridors of the hospital, in a panic.

They sensed it was over when they saw Anne in the hallway, leaning against the wall, weeping. She was standing, waiting to give them directions to where Carmen was relocated. The ongoing renovations in the hospital make it difficult to find your way.

Denise is first to reach Anne. "Is she gone?" she asks as Anne jumps into her arms.

Softly Anne responds, "Yes."

"NO! NO! NO!" Denise cries, "It can't be. She left the same way Dad did."

When Dad passed away Denise, Joanne and I ran into the hospital room minutes after he left. His body was still warm. We had been with him all night and went to bed shortly after lunch. Mom, David and Carmen stayed with him for the afternoon. We barely slept a few hours when we received the call. I'm convinced I drove the 30 km from Warren to Sturgeon Falls asleep or in a trance. I woke up when two boys on bikes pulled out between parked cars to cross the street right in front of my car. I abruptly slammed on the brakes barely missing them. They kept talking and pedalling oblivious to their surroundings. We were seconds from the hospital parking lot. The car dashboard clock read 4 P.M. – the time of my father's passing.

★ ★ ★

George is following behind. Anne turns her head toward the trauma room. Her nod indicates this is where Carmen is located, a few steps away. As Denise and George approach, the doors open automatically.

Carmen is lying on her back; her bed is slightly elevated from behind. As they walk in Carmen's head tilts slightly to her left side. Her jaw is open. They reach for her – they touch her – they caress her – her body is still warm.

George pulls out a Kleenex and wipes the froth from Carmen's mouth. It comes naturally to him. He strokes her hair. He caresses her face. "*Ahh, mon bébé! mon bébé!*" – he continues to tell her he loves her. And he cries. That's all he can do.

George detects a tear in the corner of Carmen's left eye. Denise watches as he wipes it; a second appears. He leaves it. This one remains intact. He describes it, "Like in a fairy tale, frozen in time, it hangs beautifully and crystallized."

Denise can't believe they did not make it in time. She lifts the blanket to look at her younger sister. Lying on her back in her hospital gown – Carmen's leg is bent in her usual position. Her stomach and chest are not moving. She is still. She is dead.

George is in denial.

Moments later, they sense Carmen's spirit in the room. They look around. They feel her presence. Her spirit becomes very prominent.

Martin and Anne walk in and out of the room. Martin makes numerous phone calls, often breaking into tears. His eyelids are red and swollen as a result, a distinct family trait. Anne's role is to give directions as people arrive.

Julie, Carmen's co-worker, and her husband Jack stayed a long time. Joanne and Ken are next to appear in the room. Denise steps out temporarily to contact Sam. Once she returns, she sees Lisa, who remains on the other side of the curtain, away from her mother's lifeless body. Someone pulled the curtain alongside Carmen's bed to create a separation.

People are moving from one side of the curtain to the other. George remains discreetly at the back next to Carmen's head, giving people the space they need while he continues to caress her. He can't leave her.

Within a few hours, Carmen's body begins to change. It is gradually getting colder; her body is stiffening and the color – a fluorescent yellow. Just like Dad.

George strokes her hair for hours until it is time to leave. Denise recalls how Carmen's hair was curly when they arrived. By the time they left, the many strokes had straightened her hair. The chemo is what made it curl. It's now back to its natural state.

The family leaves, tired and in disbelief. They go for breakfast to a local restaurant and by coincidence, Julie and Jack, who left the hospital earlier, are there. They spend a few hours together. The family then proceeds to Carmen's apartment.

It's a beautiful sunny day; Denise, Joanne and Martin take turns riding the scooter around the building. Once they are done playing with Carmen's new toy, they gather in the living room.

George is standing in front of the fireplace, transfixed by Carmen's picture sitting on the mantle. He wants a replica. Carmen is beautiful. She's in her early thirties, holding her baby Lisa in her arms.

He cries again, "I should have come to check on her earlier. I should have paid more attention to all her medication ... and her nutrition."

He feels he did not do enough. He feels he could have done more. He maintains, "She just slipped out of our hands!"

That night George sleeps in Carmen's bed. Next to him on the dresser sits the picture of his love. They spend their last night together.

Denise snores in the guest bedroom.

★ ★ ★

I lay in bed. I cannot sleep at all. My heart is broken, shattered in a million pieces. I ache. I cry. I am stressed thinking of funeral arrangements. I feel awful. I feel sick to my stomach. I could easily vomit.

My mind brings me to revisit my last conversations with my sister, our last days together. It was like a broken record, over and over again. I come to believe I abandoned my sister.

Again I wondered, my going to Toronto – was it really necessary? Could I not see the signs? And then telling her that for Thanksgiving, I may go to Mom's given Roger is off hunting. "Maybe I will go with you?" she says. I reply, "But you can't sit in the car for that long." What was I thinking? She must have felt abandoned by me. What was wrong with me? Why did I not stay with her after my trip to France? Already it was hard for her to let me go for three weeks. Did I not have enough of a break? Was golf that important? Was I scared? Did I sense it was coming?

I knew she was not feeling well. She was not calling as often that week. She had a cold that was getting worse. Her voice sounded tired. I told her she should be seeking medical attention early on for her cold. She should be going to the hospital, given that she was on chemo. She wasn't listening to my instructions. She phoned her pharmacist for cough medication instead.

When we spoke Tuesday night, Carmen argued with me again about going to the emergency but promised to see her family physician the next morning. She ended our call with a soft, "I love you sis." I followed with, "Me too sis. Sleep well." Her "Love you" sounded different that night. I reflected on it for a few minutes once we hung up. I sensed it was her last. That couldn't be. No, it couldn't be.

The next morning I phone en route to Toronto. She had just returned from her appointment with her family physician. It was pneumonia. He prescribed antibiotics. Odd, he told her he wasn't sure if he was giving her the right prescription given the chemo she was taking. She plans to rest and go ahead with her get-together that evening. "If I'm too tired, I'll go to bed and they can stay in the living room."

"Is pneumonia contagious?" I ask. She is upset by my question. I text Martin; he will contact Lisa.

That night I spoke to Denise. Carmen was sick but resting. We had a text exchange …

September 26, 2012

The eve of my sister's passing. Denise writes:

4:55 P.M. She is sick, drugged by all the medication. Let's hope tomorrow will be better. It is so sad; she wants me to visit Anne to see Lucas.

5:08 P.M She shakes a lot. Has an enormous headache.

8:26 P.M. Just returned from Anne's. I rocked and filmed baby Lucas. Carmen is sleeping in her room. I've cancelled my day tomorrow.

Denise and I spoke shortly afterwards. I was happy she was with her. My last text to her that night:

10:00 P.M. It's funny how she shares different things with each sister. Martin told me she was tired of fighting …

The television isn't working well in our hotel room. Roger asked to change rooms. I throw my cell phone in my purse. It's on vibrate. I never heard all the buzzing that night. Denise writes again:

10:33 P.M. We are off to hospital. Ambulance is coming. Will give you news later.

September 27, 2012

12:43 A.M. Carmen is very sick; she could have a heart attack. Doctor is doing a whole lot of tests her heart is not doing well.

3:26 A.M. George & I came home to rest. I called Martin, he is there with her. Will have news around 6 A.M.

I wake up at 3 A.M. I tell Roger I don't have a good feeling about Carmen. I want to return home first thing in the morning. An hour or so later I charge my cell. For the first time, I see Denise's messages. I had a few from Martin as well.

1:30 A.M. My mom is in the hospital.

1:31 A.M. Her heart is very weak.

Roger and I leave Toronto immediately.

★ ★ ★

The morning following my sister's passing, Roger suggests I ask her for forgiveness. I do so. I think I feel better.

Most of the week is chaotic, so many details to look after; the loss is sickening; the demands from individuals are taxing; the fatigue is accumulating; and my brain is not functioning. I cannot concentrate. I am not sleeping. Everything seems to take much longer: finalizing arrangements with the funeral home, the cemetery, the flowers, etc. I struggle to write the obituary – I can't see the words. I only see letters.

The small stuff is stressful; the devil is in the detail. I don't want this responsibility. Where is everybody? I too want to sit back and look at family pictures.

I am only able to relax the eve of the funeral when all is practically ready. With the funeral arrangements et al, we are out of the house for hours at a time. I don't recall what everyone else was doing, but people were busy. My nephew Patrick is assembling a slide presentation of precious photos for the wake. I focus on the funeral with Martin and George; Roger, Mom and Tim focus on everything else. The house will be full.

My Uncle Denis phoned several times. We keep missing his calls. Had we not been so busy and heartbroken and in an unusual state of mind, we would have been happy to help him out with his many questions, ranging from hotel accommodations, to which road he should take to come up and the location of the service.

I feel my mother's discomfort with respect to our cousin. Jennifer inquires if she is welcome to attend the funeral. Strange, I thought. Why would someone not be welcome at a funeral? I refused to go there. I assign that one to my mother, "You deal with it Mom."

Planning a funeral is difficult. You are grieving. Some people question your decisions until you clarify that, "These are her wishes, not mine. Decisions she made before leaving." One has little energy to meet everyone's needs when your world is falling apart.

We are very pleased to see everyone. They too are grieving. Grief makes us all behave in strange ways.

Throughout the ordeal, we drop in at Carmen's to seek comfort in her apartment. I feel she is with us throughout the week. The family is together.

October 2, 2012
It was a gorgeous day - the start of the fall foliage - temperature was 25C. I report to Louise, Carmen's friend, who could not be with us.

> "Carmen had the nicest funeral – the flowers, the urn, the room overflowing with family and friends – we were missing chairs. The priest gave a warm and personal service. The eulogy was very touching. It was written and delivered by Anne, Martin's new girlfriend."

> "The family met at my place after the cemetery. At the end of the evening, Martin asked Anne for her hand in marriage. The wedding will be held in Cuba. Carmen would be so proud of him. I know we are."

> "Although certain moments were difficult, it was a beautiful and peaceful day."

At home the night of the funeral, David takes me aside, hugs me and thanks me for everything I did for Carmen. I appreciate that. It means a lot to me. I know I heard thank you from others throughout the year but this one resonates more, probably because our journey is over and I am listening.

THE AFTERMATH

A few days later, I realize Carmen passed away on the same day Dad was buried; September 27. She kept a connection with him. She had previously mentioned to me that she did not want to die on the same day he did; September 24.

My father passed away at the age of 73; he quit smoking five years before his diagnosis. Carmen was 60; she quit four years before hers.

Smoking causes lung cancer and more. Losing someone you love is difficult, but seeing them suffer is painful and heartbreaking. We have four smokers in the family; we all wish they would quit. What is it we don't understand?

The Saturday after her funeral, George and I begin liquidating Carmen's apartment. We sort through all her belongings, making piles for the needy, piles to discard. It's important for us to donate what we can, out of respect for my sister. We put in full days. It takes time. Every item brings memories. We individually reflect on everything we touch … this was her favorite sweater … she bought this in … I gave her this … we do it for Carmen. Does it help our grieving? I'm not sure. It does bring more emotions to the surface. We don't know what her children want to keep. "No. Don't want it," is a typical reply.

The siblings and Mom request a personal souvenir of Carmen. Nothing cries out, "Take me – take me!" I conclude my sister is somewhat of a hoarder. I reflect on my own home. I must clean my house; otherwise, my executor will never be done.

I continue to triage my sister's clothes. I'm emptying a hamper in her bedroom closet. I toss a few more blouses in the charity pile. As I pick up a sweater, I see a mason jar hidden in the basket. I can't make out the contents. It looks like body parts, an off-white colour. I'm baffled. I pick it up. I still can't figure out the contents. I walk to the window for better light. I unscrew the jar and the smell of nicotine reaches my nostrils. I pull out a piece of damp cream-coloured Kleenex. I unroll it to find a cigarette butt; half the cigarette had been smoked. I unroll the others – the same. I count 10. All Du Maurier. This used to be my father's brand but not my sister's. I return them to the jar and call for George. He's cleaning another room. He's as surprised as I am to see this. He's upset. "Someone has given her cigarettes while I spent the year, day and night, trying to save her life. Who could have done this?"

We make our way outside to the terrace to find the smokers' can ashtray. We go through all the butts. I'm happy not to find a Du Maurier.

We don't know if someone gave her the cigarettes or if she took them from someone's pack. We do not pursue the investigation. What would be the purpose? I leave the jar on the shelf for her children to find.

I still can't understand why she kept them. She knew we would find them. Why did she not flush them down the toilet? She wanted us to know. Was the nicotine addiction that strong to lure her back? Did she want to accelerate her death? It explains the odd tobacco smell in the kitchen, the strong odour of Lestoil to disguise it, and the small lighter we found the same day in her bedroom.

I come across my old silver charm bracelet. One I used to wear when I was 15. I thought I had discarded it. Odd, she kept this. It reminds me of my letters, the ones I wrote 40 years ago. I search for them. I can't find them. Where have they gone?

More than one week goes by; still George and I are the only two working in the apartment. It seems it is expected. Where is the rest of the family? More than 95% of the work is done. I find it upsetting. I decide not to take the lead any longer. I leave her children a list of what is sold; tell them what is left to do. It took them an afternoon to discard the rest. They set aside a box of souvenirs for us to go through.

Roger, George and I return to pick up the remaining items. We clean the apartment. It's ready for the next tenant. The computer and printer are the only items remaining.

I take home a box of books I was expecting her children to discard. Books on healthy eating habits, death and dying, healing and angels; all I'm convinced my sister barely or never read. Books I shall read.

I don't understand my feelings. I'm somewhat angry or maybe it's disappointment, I'm not quite sure ... and I don't know why ... and I don't know towards whom. Am I angry at myself for taking all the responsibility again? Am I angry at myself for not being wiser ... for not providing better emotional support? Am I upset for not being there ... at Carmen for not sharing ... at myself for not asking ... at others, for moving on? I need yoga. I need meditation. I need to get my shit together.

I text my siblings, "If you want to hear Carmen's voice one last time, you need to call her number today. Her phone will be disconnected tomorrow. A new tenant is coming in." David cried when he heard Carmen's voice mail message. She had a beautiful voice.

★ ★ ★

"When I miss her the most I have dreams," reveals Lisa.

In all her dreams, Lisa realizes her mother could leave anytime, any minute. Although she doesn't sleep well, Lisa feels better the next day. She heard her mother's voice in her dreams – it was truly her voice. In a sense she found it comforting having extra time with her mom.

> "I feel so blessed I can see my mom in my dreams and so far they were all good dreams. She tries to make me feel better. The book I'm reading, *The Wheel of Life*, is really good and has changed my thinking about my mom being gone. Funny thing in most of my dreams I'm always talking to my mom on the phone, maybe she really wants me to know it's her, so we talk on the phone, lol."

We lived the past year knowing Carmen would be leaving us. Sometimes Lisa continues to live it in her dreams. The formal farewell, the waving of the hand, the whisper of the word "goodbye" does not happen at the moment one departs for the next world. Instead, it is expressed repeatedly through our gestures, our choices, our compassion, our care and our love, as we progress through this journey together.

On occasion, Lisa sees Lucas laugh and smile at nothing. She wonders – does he see Carmen in the room? "Are you smiling at grand-maman? Is she there with you?"

The different stages of grieving come and go in waves; for some, it's dealing with emptiness; for others, it remains surreal. We move on but she is still with us. I like to think she's just in the other room. At times I wonder how she is.

"Sometimes I feel my mother's spirit. Sometimes I ask her for help." Martin recalls looking for an important document for his mother's estate. He could not find it. He knew he left it in Anne's condo but he couldn't find it. It could not be at his mother's; the only remaining items are the computer and printer. In tears, he asks his mom for help. He later went to Carmen's apartment. He loads the computer and keyboard into his van. As he picks up the printer he hears something fall ... it's the document he was looking for. "It was impossible for it to be there, I distinctly remember bringing it to Anne's condo." Carmen becomes his new St. Anthony of Padua.

Carmen chose to leave when her two children had a new and deepest love in their lives. Martin is head over heels in love with Anne, and Lisa with her new baby, Lucas.

The Sunday following the funeral, Denise attends mass in her parish in Saint-Sauveur. The priest informs all parishioners, "Be careful when walking in the cemetery. A bear cub has been spotted in the last few days. The mother bear has not been seen." Denise looks in astonishment. Tinour?

A week later, I'm golfing with a friend. We are on the back nine at Eagle Creek Golf Club; I'm looking in my bag and can't find my five iron. I know I used it that day on a previous hole. Natalie and I both go through my golf bag, looking at every club. Not there. I ask her to check her own bag in case I dropped it in hers by mistake. Not there. I play my six iron and end up short of the green in the sand trap. I comment on my shot while looking at Natalie. I turn around as I begin to walk, and there it is – my five iron – sticking out as if someone had partly pulled it out of my golf bag. I immediately thought of my sister.

★ ★ ★

I've only had the one dream.

"What are you doing?" I ask as I lay in bed in the middle of the night, my eyes closed. I feel my sister's presence. She is very close to me.

"I'm waiting," she says.

"Waiting for what?"

"I see two doors."

★ ★ ★

I receive a text from Lisa.

> "My friend Jody that got in vitro done, is pregnant :) My mom told her she had a direct line with God and she was going make it happen. She kept her word :) Her baby is due end of July, beginning of August."

Carmen's birthday is August 1st. When Jody heard the news, she immediately looked up at the sky and said, "Thank you Mom!" Meaning, thank you Carmen. Lisa's closest friends always called her mother "Mom". The couple had been trying for years. Their dream is finally coming true.

As I finalize my book and consider my options for publication, I decide to contact Lori Hope the author of *Help me live* to obtain permission to reproduce parts of her work. I Google her name to find her website. To my surprise, she has passed away. The first item listed by Google is her obituary. I read it in sadness and read it again. I am taken aback when I realize she passed away on September 27, 2012, the same day as Carmen. She was diagnosed with advanced lung cancer the summer of 2011. The two had a parallel journey. I am shaken up by the news. I feel a strong connection to Lori Hope.

I wonder if they met at the gates. They must have. My sister loved her book. She probably asked her for her autograph.

Mystical experiences, do they exist?

To the few examples you read earlier in my book, I add the following.

Carmen has been speaking to me in different ways. I know she is responsible for leaving certain books in my path. Books that help me and other family members understand that dying is part of living and that there is life after death. Books that remind us of the purpose of life.

I don't recall the exact words that brought me her message but as I'm reading *Wheel of Life* by Dr. Elisabeth Kübler-Ross, toward the end of the book I sense my sister telling me, "There is a God. There is life after death." Her message shakes me.

Do you see dead people before you die?

Our Great Aunt Lora did during her final days. Carmen asked the same question. The day before she left us, she told Denise she saw Ron and a lot of people she did not know. Could they have been her angels?

At the very beginning of his journey, my father had terrible nightmares. He only shared a few details – people he did not know, an ugly scene, forks and shovels. As he progressed in his journey the nightmares disappeared. He was at peace.

What about a bright light?

Two of my uncles claimed they saw one before being revived; Tom, in the hospital after a heart attack; Claude, after a major car accident.

Marie shared with us that she saw a bright white hand reach for her, she grabbed it and then let go. She wasn't ready. This was after a major car accident, a few years before her cancer diagnosis.

Can you feel a presence, a spirit?

When my father died, we all felt his presence in the room even more so than when he was alive. The family stayed in the hospital room with him for more than two hours after he passed. His presence was warm and peaceful.

Those present could feel Carmen's spirit in the trauma room after her passing. Roger and I did not. She wasn't with us in the morgue that day, not in spirit. I wish I had felt her presence. I wonder if it would be easier to let go.

Close friends of ours lost a son unexpectedly at a young age. His spirit was present in their house for close to one year, until the parents were finally able to bring some closure. Today they communicate through a medium.

In 2010, I encountered a spirit while walking the Camino de Santiago, a pilgrimage route in Spain. Denise and I were spending the night in a hotel in Sarria. We left the window open for the fresh night air. Denise was sleeping. I was reading a suspense novel and couldn't put it down.

It was late at night when I felt the spirit enter the room. His presence made me feel tense; I felt a pressure in my chest. I could feel this negative energy. I remember asking myself – should I close the window? I continued reading my book, hoping it would go away. I get ready for bed. I'm still uncomfortable. I proceed to turn off the lights and notice Denise is not snoring – unusual. I could still feel this presence. I focus on my breath – my yoga breath – deep inhale; slow exhale to calm myself. The window and the curtains remain open. The street light provides just enough light for me to see Denise in her bed. Minutes pass. She's still not snoring. She's sleeping on her right side; her back to me.

I hear this deep voice coming from her body – animal like – incomprehensible. It reminds me of the exorcist. I quickly sit in my bed and scream, "DENISE? WHAT ARE YOU DOING?" She turns over to face me. She never woke up. I'm not sure what to do. I lay in bed staring at her. Her breathing is shallow. Her chest rises and falls rapidly with every breath. Finally, I feel the spirit leave the room. The window remains open and eventually I fall asleep.

The next morning I chose not to discuss it with Denise for fear she may think she's possessed. We begin our walk early as usual and stop for coffee at the next village. At breakfast she shares her nightmare, "Someone was trying to kill me." She did not seem surprised when I told her my experience. She replies, "I could hear someone calling my name during my dream, but from afar." That was the only spirit we encountered on the Camino. Thank God.

★ ★ ★

I have a much better appreciation today of what my father was living when he was dying of cancer. I am more knowledgeable. Sharing his journey brought the family together. The word "love" became part of our vocabulary. My dad's wish was for us to stay united as a family. As a result, we are much closer today. His death was an initiation for us. He prepared us for Carmen's journey.

At times, I thought the load was heavy. Everyone does what they can. Everyone has to be comfortable with the support they provide. Now that she is gone, I wish I had done more, although at the time, I thought I did as much as I could. It was the same for my dad. I was too tired the last month to drive back up north on weekends. I remember crying days before he died, "I can't take this anymore." I never understood where George and my mother found the energy to be full-time caregivers. They never complained about their role. Thank God they were there.

Months have gone by and I have never felt worse physically in my entire life. I believe it is the mourning, the accumulated stress of the past year and the weight gain. I quit drinking coffee (but not wine); I feel a difference in my nervous system. I promise myself to pursue a healthier and more balanced lifestyle, one with good eating habits, exercise, yoga, meditation — activities that will improve my physical and mental state. My second promise is to move forward from the planning to the execution stage.

We are adjusting to a new landscape. The communication between family members has greatly diminished since my sister's passing. People are moving on, getting back to their routines. The family dynamics have changed. The missing link is the communicator. Carmen was that central figure. The one who knew what everyone else was up to. Carmen was the one who contacted us all on a regular basis. She kept us together.

To remain united as a family will require an effort, but it's a promise worth keeping.

WRITING THIS BOOK

I've been crying for weeks, and more. I try to write but I can barely see my computer screen. The tears come down in buckets. Ironically, the email that torments me becomes the email that saves me, "… it is better to get it off your chest than to keep it bottled inside." Carmen is speaking to me and I cannot hear; I cannot see. I am lost – too focused on my mourning.

Writing my introduction came effortlessly. The words and tears just flowed naturally. Am I crazy to do this? Am I experiencing an emotional breakdown writing this book? I want people to know how it feels but it's not like me to share my vulnerability. I seek external validation. I forwarded a copy of my introduction to a few family members and friends. It eventually brings me to draft my conclusion at which time I realize I am getting better. My sister is guiding me and has been throughout this entire exercise.

There are so many great authors and very knowledgeable people on topics related to death and dying. I'm not one of them. I'm an individual who has lost a few people she loves and who will most likely experience it again, unless of course, I'm next.

When I began writing this book, my initial goal was to raise awareness on end-of-life issues. I didn't want to focus solely on the challenges but also on the opportunities to share precious moments with loved ones. At times I felt I was not well equipped to care for my sister. Today I realize that I may have been more critical of myself than I should have been. Although I was not with her for her last breath, I supported her the best I could throughout her journey. We all did. We were all there for her. Each person brought something special. Carmen did not die alone.

There are many more stories and events from our last year together. Some repetitious; some forgotten; some will come to mind once this book is published; and of course, other perspectives.

The following was the last chapter left for me to summarize. Thinking it was repetitious, I never sent it to my family. Today, I share it for it is more relevant than ever. I like to think these are my sister's last words.

Help me live: Chapter 21 – "I am more grateful than I can say for your care, compassion, and support."

- I will forever be grateful – they helped me live.
- Our biggest fear is that people won't be there for us when we need them most – and when we have cancer, we regress to a state of dependency and thus need people more than most. Our greatest hope is that they will show up.
- I would never wish such trauma on anyone, but if ever you are lost in terror, grief, or hopelessness, I hope you will be able to mouth these words yourself "I am more grateful than I can say for your care, compassion and support."
- Please forgive us if we forget to say thank you. Sometimes we don't have the energy and have to break the cardinal rule of manners.

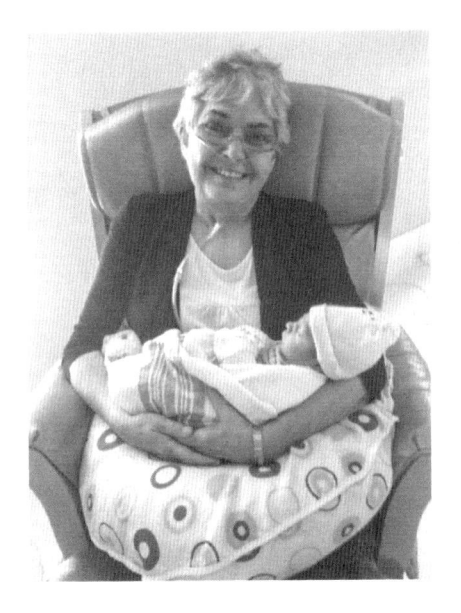

My sister Carmen and her first grandson Lucas September 12, 2012. The photo was taken shortly after a chemo treatment two weeks prior to her passing. Lucas was barely eight hours old. She was his first visitor.

A THANK YOU LETTER TO GEORGE

George has graciously given me permission to share this special letter with you.

To my love George,
How can I ever thank you for everything you have done? It's impossible. Thank you cannot begin to express my gratitude for all you do for me. Where would I be if you were not here? Without a doubt my health would be worse. You have done so much for me and my family. I apologize for my mood swings, for my demands and for making you so nervous. Thank you for remaining calm. I wanted us to go away for a few days but it hasn't worked out. I hope we can do so shortly if my health will permit.

I know you tell me it's because you want me cured and sometimes it makes me impatient but I do listen and I hear you. I am a prisoner of my body. Sometimes I think renting a room in a seniors residence would be best. We don't know when I will need care 24 hours a day. I would like to discuss it with you. It would give everyone a break, especially yourself. I don't want you to burn out.

We have been together for so long. The kids consider you their father and I know you love them as your own. I know you will always be there for them and especially my grandchildren. You are their only grandfather so you must hug and kiss them for both of us. You must attend all family gatherings because you are family. We are your family and we all love you. Hold on to our fond memories and share them with the family; especially my little ones to come. Don't forget, you can call them once a week!

Never will I ever be able to repay you for everything you do for me. Although sometimes I may not show it or say it, I am more grateful than you know. I thank you a thousand times for taking care of me.

I love you, Carmen.

CONCLUSION

I'm not sure what was more painful: my sister's passing on September 27, 2012 or learning she had terminal lung cancer a year earlier. My heart ached for her from the very beginning.

There are many facets of a terminal illness for both the patient and the caregivers. It's an ongoing, intense learning experience for all and a unique journey for each. Our new "normal" becomes the unknown, the turbulence of intense and powerful emotions, the isolation, the helplessness, the bouts of depression, the waves of mourning; it goes on. We live in a different world. Our surroundings are foreign.

Deep within us, we choose to find the courage. We open our hearts, together we become vulnerable, we cry, we laugh, we give, we receive, we forgive, we support, we don't understand and eventually, we accept. Is there a better expression of love? This journey gave our family the opportunity to choose love, to care for and to appreciate one another.

The greatest gift we could give my sister was to be by her side during the most traumatic time in her life. The most beautiful gift Carmen could give us was to allow us to share our love.

Every family has its own challenges. Can one grow without pain? What lessons remain? Somewhere along the way we stopped resisting. The disappearance of my brother Robert left us speculating and without closure. To this day, we don't know if he is alive. The passing of my dad brought us closer, Carmen's even more. At times, I worry another one of us will go shortly, before I have time to heal. My heart remains tender and raw. I realize I need to be patient and give time, time.

Does it get easier with experience? I wonder. Do we eventually become habituated to death?

I have the utmost respect for my sister – for her courage, her generosity, her simplicity and for the non-materialistic person she was. I hold the same for my dad. For both shared with us their journey to peace. Both had strength of character I had not imagined. Both are in a much better place somewhere in this Universe.

I take away many lessons, some of which I don't fully comprehend. I'm slowly coming back to earth, my feet not yet touching the ground. I hope when they do I will understand.

Every death is different and every journey unique. I wish we (an all inclusive we) had a better understanding of end-of-life care in all aspects. I wish we had a better appreciation of the value we bring to a stranger or to a loved one throughout their final journey.

A friend once told me, "I cry for you and for all who have shared a similar experience and loss."

I cry for those who experience this alone. Every life is precious. What matters most is to love and to be loved.

No one wants to die, alone.

SPECIAL CONTRIBUTION

By Ariane de Bonvoisin, Change expert

I've been exploring the subject of life changes for many years. I have written books and articles intended to help people navigate both the beautiful and the heart breaking changes that come our way and have helped people individually and in groups. I do not claim to be an expert in any specific change, as each is so incredibly personal. What I have been privileged to see, is what helps some people during transitional times, and why they get through change and others stay in pain or paralysis for years. I have referred to these in my work as " The 9 Principles of Change."

There are no words, written or spoken that can really help someone who is faced with an illness such as cancer, or for the friends and family that surround that person and will see them pass on. Changes of this sort are the most difficult we will ever face. They will define us. In the end, they are always an invitation to pause, focus on what is essential, to go inside to find what matters and not to our busy external lives, and to make a choice on how to live. While the mind will often go to "What to do?" under these painful circumstances the question at the start is always "How to be?"

That, we have control over.

People who get through changes of all kinds have the following common characteristics, which I humbly invite you to consider:

They are optimists. They have positive beliefs about themselves, other people, and life in general. They do not act or feel like victims, there is no energy of poor-me. They live in a friendly world, not a dangerous or fearful one. They remain open-minded to solutions, to any type of help that might show up. They are present, not living overly in the past or the future. They are nice, solid people to be around. They exude positive energy. We all know these types of people.

They believe and live what I call 'The Change Guarantee': *From this change, something good will come.* This isn't easy to see in the midst of pain and extreme grief, but with time, and with a focus on this as being true, what is good and beautiful post this change, will reveal itself. It may come in the form of renewed faith in something greater, improved relationships, forgiveness, better health habits, a new career or a surprise of some sort, starting a foundation to help others, or simply becoming more like the person you were meant to be.

People who are able to handle any change remember they have a "Change Muscle". We are all so much better at change than we have ever been told, we are resilient and need to be reminded that we have and will continue to face changes of all sorts with immense courage.

When tough changes arrive, we are thrown into very difficult emotions; fear, doubt, sadness, guilt, blame, anger… People who are good at change are very human; they feel their emotions deeply. They do not hide out in being strong or in their full to-do lists. They are vulnerable. They allow any emotion to be present; they feel it fully until it passes. They go to the anti-dote of that emotion, for example, from fear to faith, from doubt to surrender, from guilt to forgiveness.

Resistance to the change is what causes so much pain. As impossible as it first appears, acceptance of what life has now handed, is the remedy. We always lose when we argue with reality. This principle of change is one of Acceptance. It takes time. And it does come. Be prepared for the person to change radically - physically, emotionally and mentally. Their life view, their faith, what they want to do or not do now may change. This can be very hard to accept but is necessary. It will help them let go if they feel loved and accepted despite how different they are becoming.

When change knocks, we feel out of control. So it is helpful to ask, what can I control? It is never anything on the outside, no people, no circumstances, and definitely not time itself. You can control the questions you ask yourself (e.g. instead of Why is this happening? try, How can I show up positively for this person?), the language you use (instead of using words like disaster, tragedy…try words like challenge or experience). The stories you tell yourself and others now about this change and your overall mindset are also under your control. You can be a warning or an example for how to be. Do not bring your worry or anxiety energy to this person.

They will feel it. It is better for you to go and take care of yourself if you find you are in this space. Come back when you are ready. You may also notice that you desperately want to take control over something - doing the dishes, cleaning up, watering the garden, changing your tires etc. Just be aware that although some of these can be helpful, it is often the mind trying to get some sense of certainty in the face of radical uncertainty.

All change is an invitation to find our spiritual self, our Higher Self, the part of us that is unchangeable, eternal, all knowing, in touch with something beyond words. When everything around you is in flux, people who find that inner peace are able to find a strength that is larger than their own. Faith of any kind, whether it is Grace, God, Buddha, Divine Mother, Allah, The Universe… is one of the pillars of people who get through change. Most faiths talk of something beautiful after death, something eternal, beyond the body, which renews the hope of something good happening in the future.

No one goes through a change like cancer or losing a loved one alone. And yet, we often feel like we are the only person going through this, the only one to cry as much, to feel so lost, so finished. The people you surround yourself have a huge influence on how you feel when faced with change. Make sure you have a great change support team. Many times, life brings you new people to help. Don't expect your closest friends to be there for you. Sometimes you may be surprised at who shows up and also who doesn't. Let it be. Everyone is facing their pain in the only way they know how. And remember; ask for what you need. If you need a cooked meal, ask for it.

Finally, while change is certainly an emotional journey first and foremost, there are some actions to take, regardless of circumstances. The number one thing to often go out the window when you go through change is your health. You sleep less, you eat less or more, you often drink more (coffee, alcohol), and you stop exercising. And so, your capacity to have energy and reserves is far diminished. You show up empty for the person you are caring for. Taking care of yourself and specifically your health, (remember the acronym S.E.E.D - Sleep, Exercise, Eat well, Drink water), should be top of the list. It is an act of love and high self-esteem and also the best way to build courage for the journey ahead. If you do not, there is a knock on effect on the rest of your life; your kids, your job etc.

suffer. Plus, any form of exercise will help move all the tough emotions that show up out of you, instead of stacking them away somewhere in the body. You must take care of your needs as well. And that includes resting. Yes, that can be very confronting because when you rest, it is often when your emotions catch up with you.

I've witnessed many friends lose a family member or friend to cancer and other diseases. What I have noticed is that all agree on spending some time on the basics that need to be taken care of. As hard as it is to have a conversation with someone about preparing for what is to come, you never want to give up the fight and admit the inevitable is going to happen. You never know if your loved one has a week, a month or a year left, so take the time to ask questions about bank accounts, passwords, finances, transferring titles & things into other people's names early on. After someone passes, people spend so much time trying to sort out financial issues. This becomes their focus instead of being with the loss and celebrating the person's life.

No matter what job you have, nothing matters more than spending time with a loved one as they're fighting cancer (or any life threatening illness). Most people I've spoken to all wish they had spent more time with their loved one.

This is really a somber thought, but have a conversation about how and where they want their funeral. Details, songs, people, special things will mean a lot to them and to you when the day comes.

Finally, it is important to remember your other roles, despite being there for the person who has cancer. You may be a parent, a grandparent, a sibling, a friend, a spouse, a colleague etc. All these people still need you in some small way. Your life can feel meaningless now in the face of your coming loss. Details seem irrelevant. The person who is facing cancer wants you to continue your life. It helps them in some way to know that life hasn't changed that much. They do not want to be seen or ever feel like a sacrifice. Come back to their side with stories, what happened in your day, humor, even sharing with them your challenges, what you need help on. Don't think your stuff is too small. Include them. You are still human. You still have everyday challenges. Don't suddenly pretend around them that your whole life is fine.

Be fiercely determined to be what I call a *'change optimist'*: someone who can both feel the pain of this journey through cancer, and also someone who will find their way, bounce back and take everyone else with them.

Nicole is certainly one of these people and I honor her for what she has been a witness to and also how she has come to embody the change guarantee. Thanks to what she went through, this profound wisdom is now being shared with others through this wonderful book.

Blessings and love on your journey,
Ariane

Ariane de Bonvoisin is an author, speaker, entrepreneur and change expert. Her websites can be found at www.arianedebonvoisin.com and www.first30days.com

AFTERWORD

I am blessed and fortunate to have the love and support of so many wonderful people. Through this initiative, I've received assistance from individuals who want to make this world a better place – people who want to better humanity. I call each one a friend.

To quote Ariane from her work "The Change Guarantee: From this change, something good will come." I imagine a more compassionate community where families are better prepared to support their loved one; where health care professionals have access to resources to enhance their skill set and better support their patients.

As faith would have it, in finalizing this memoir I discovered a unique coaching program in my city. The Ottawa Regional Cancer Foundation (ORCF) initiated a cancer-coaching program using a solution-focused and person-centred approach. Their mission is to empower individuals affected by cancer – patients and caregivers – and to engage the survivor in his or her own care.

This program is a gem on many fronts – from a revolutionary cancer coaching model to the dedicated and committed professionals focusing on an individual's needs – physical, informational, emotional and spiritual – to help them meet the challenges of cancer and live well.

Cancer coaching is a new concept in cancer care. Still in its nascent phase this program needs the financial resources to continue to thrive and expand. It needs our support.

Making a difference

Until a cure for cancer is found help the ORCF address the needs of survivors and their families … help them create an innovative best practice coaching program for those affected by cancer – the first of its kind in Canada. Help them help you – your loved ones – your friends – your neighbours.

Please join me in supporting the ORCF. I thank you in advance for your generous donation. I thank you for sharing my story.

I wish you health. I wish you love. Nicole

To learn more about the great things the ORCF does – visit www.ottawacancer.ca

OTTAWA REGIONAL CANCER FOUNDATION
1500 Alta Vista Drive Ottawa | Ontario | K1G 3Y9
PHONE: 613.247.3527 TOLL FREE: 1.855.247.3527

OTHER READINGS

The following books and resources are ones I found most informative and helpful in guiding us in our journey. I encourage you to read on the subject and benefit from the unique experience of others. I hope my book serves you in the same way.

Help Me Live, Revised: 20 Things People with Cancer Want You to Know
By Lori Hope
The author was a cancer survivor who surveyed 600 patients. Targeted to family, friends and cancer survivors, this insightful book provides clarification on patients' feelings and thoughts. You consciously develop your list of do's and don'ts.

Saying Goodbye: A Guide to Coping with a Loved One's Terminal Illness
By Barbara Okun, Ph.D. and Joseph Nowinski, Ph.D.
The book introduces you to the changing face of grief as patients' survival times are prolonged due to medical advancement. It guides you through the five stages of family grief and helps you understand what to expect and how to prepare.

The Wheel of Life
By Dr. Elisabeth Kübler-Ross
A well-known author, medical doctor and psychiatrist, she tells the story of her extraordinary life. The book speaks of her research on death and life after death. It may help you understand and accept that dying is part of life.

On Death and Dying
By Dr. Elisabeth Kübler-Ross
As one of the foremost authorities on death and dying, in this book she explored the five stages of death. You gain a better understanding of how imminent death affects patients.

The Canadian Virtual Hospice
www.virtualhospice.ca
This site is an excellent resource. It provides information and support on palliative and end-of-life care, loss and grief. You can contact their team of professionals for answers to your personal questions on terminal illness and loss.

The First 30 Days: Your Guide to Making Any Change Easier
By Ariane de Bonvoisin
I read this book after completing my manuscript. The author, a change expert, introduces "The 9 Principles of Change" and describes how some people successfully manage change. I was amazed how I could easily identify each principle in my book as I went through this major loss in my life. Being aware of the principles may help you better reflect on your own situation and help you navigate through these difficult times. Visit www.arianedebonvoisin.com and www.first30days.com

Printed in Canada